SKIN LONGEVITY SECRETS UNVEILED

DISCOVER HOW ANYONE CAN ACHIEVE TIMELESS BEAUTY, RADIANT SKIN, AND REDUCE WRINKLES AND FINE LINES WITHOUT SURGERY

AGELESS REVELATIONS

© **Copyright 2024 - All rights reserved.**

The content contained within this book may not be reproduced, duplicated or transmitted without direct written permission from the author or the publisher.

Under no circumstances will any blame or legal responsibility be held against the publisher, or author, for any damages, reparation, or monetary loss due to the information contained within this book, either directly or indirectly.

Legal Notice:

This book is copyright protected. It is only for personal use. You cannot amend, distribute, sell, use, quote or paraphrase any part, or the content within this book, without the consent of the author or publisher.

Disclaimer Notice:

Please note the information contained within this document is for educational and entertainment purposes only. All effort has been executed to present accurate, up to date, reliable, complete information. No warranties of any kind are declared or implied. Readers acknowledge that the author is not engaged in the rendering of legal, financial, medical or professional advice. The content within this book has been derived from various sources. Please consult a licensed professional before attempting any techniques outlined in this book.

By reading this document, the reader agrees that under no circumstances is the author responsible for any losses, direct or indirect, that are incurred as a result of the use of the information contained within this document, including, but not limited to, errors, omissions, or inaccuracies.

CONTENTS

Introduction: Your Journey to Radiant Skin	7
1. DECODING THE SCIENCE OF AGELESS SKIN	11
The Marvel of Skin—Its Layers and Functions	12
Skin Anatomy and Recent Advancements	15
Understanding How Skin Ages	16
The Causes of Skin Aging	18
Role of Genes in Skin Aging	19
Summary	21
Segue	22
2. NOURISHING YOUR SKIN FROM WITHIN	23
A Deep Dive Into Skin-Friendly Nutrients	24
Essential Minerals	26
Antioxidants vs Free Radicals	28
Hydration and Skin Elasticity	31
The Anti-inflammatory Diet for Glowing Skin	35
Kickstart Your Glow: A Sample Anti-inflammatory Meal Plan	38
Summary	40
Segue	40
3. LIFESTYLE FACTORS AND SKIN AGING	41
How Smoking Steals Your Skin's Glow	42
Alcohol—Dehydration Party Crasher for Your Skin!	45
Feeling Stressed? It Shows on Your Skin!	47
Beauty Sleep and Skin	49
How to Catch Those Beauty Zzz	51
Summary	53
Segue	53
4. GET TO KNOW YOUR SKIN BETTER	55
Building a Personalized Skincare Routine	55
Importance of Skincare Routine	57
The Essential Steps of Your Personalized Skincare Routine	58
Morning and Night—Your Personalized Skincare Rituals Unlocked!	63

Sun Protection	64
Picking Your Perfect Sunscreen	66
Natural vs Organic Skincare	67
Three Easy DIY Recipes: Whip Up Your Own Natural Skincare	69
Summary	71
Segue	72
5. SCULPTING BEAUTY WITH FACIAL EXERCISES	**75**
Basics of Facial Exercise	76
Advantages of Facial Exercises	76
Getting Started	77
Facial Exercises	78
Creating a Routine	84
Summary	85
Segue	85
6. ADVANCED ANTI-AGING TECHNIQUES	**87**
Laser Therapy	87
Scientific Information Highlighting Emerging Trends and Innovations in Laser Treatments	89
Targeted Skin Concerns	90
Potential Side Effects	92
Before and After the Procedure	93
Aftercare for Optimized Results	94
Sharon's Story	95
Chemical Peels	96
Botox for Wrinkle Reduction	99
Dermal Fillers for Volume Restoration	101
Summary	104
Segue	105
7. EMBRACING NATURAL BEAUTY	**107**
Who Are You?	108
The Science Behind Self-Acceptance	109
Cultivating Self-Acceptance	110
Building Self-Confidence	111
Enhancing Natural Features With Makeup	112
Contouring Techniques	113
Natural Makeup Look	117
Simple Everyday Makeup Routine	118
Summary	120
Segue	120

8. PROTECTING YOUR SKIN FOR THE LONG HAUL	121
Routine Skin Check-Ups	122
How to Perform a Self-Examination	122
When to Seek Professional Help	123
Skin Cancer Prevention	124
Environmental Protection	126
Summary	128
Segue	128
9. MENTAL WELL-BEING AND TIMELESS BEAUTY	129
The Connection Between Mind and Skin	129
Managing Stress for Healthier Skin	130
Emotional Resilience and Beauty	131
Integrating Mental Wellness Into Skincare Routines	132
Summary	133
Conclusion	135
Glossary	139
References	141

INTRODUCTION: YOUR JOURNEY TO RADIANT SKIN

Have you ever looked intently in the mirror in the morning and noticed a wrinkle that you swear wasn't there the day before? Maybe you have spent a small fortune on the latest skincare products, hoping for a miracle, but still find yourself with a dull complexion staring back at you. Or perhaps you are overwhelmed and confused by the sheer volume of skincare advice available online, and you're not sure what really works. You desire that natural radiance that speaks of inner health and timeless beauty, but navigating the world of skincare can feel like a frustrating maze.

We have all experienced the desire for healthy and glowing skin, which isn't just about vanity, but also about feeling confident and comfortable in our own presence. However, the beauty industry is a multi-billion dollar machine that produces endless products and conflicting information, making anyone feel lost and defeated.

You might have tried every hack you could find online, such as DIY masks made from kitchen staples, ten-step Korean skincare routines, or overnight miracle solutions endorsed by celebrities. Nevertheless, the results are usually underwhelming, or worse, leave your skin irritated and sensitive. You are tired of being bombarded with empty promises and frustrated with the lack of real, long-term solutions. The constant barrage of conflicting advice leaves you wondering if there is a better way.

There is great news—you definitely can achieve healthy, radiant skin at any age with the secrets to skin longevity that this book unlocks. In the past, I was lost in a maze of misinformation and ineffective products, and my once vibrant skin began to show the signs of aging, making me feel unsure and self-conscious. However, I refused to accept a future of wrinkles and dullness and embarked on a journey to uncover the secrets to truly healthy, radiant skin.

What I discovered was a wealth of knowledge, combining cutting-edge science, time-tested practices, and holistic skincare approaches. This book condenses years of research, experimentation, and expert consultations into an easy-to-understand and implement comprehensive guide.

Imagine starting each day with skin that is healthy, soft, and supple, radiating a beautiful glow. Picture feeling confident and comfortable in your own skin, no matter your age. This guidebook will lead you toward achieving that reality.

Countless people, from regular folks to celebrities such as Halle Berry and Jennifer Lopez, have adopted a holistic approach to skincare and experienced remarkable transformations. These women haven't found a way to stave off the aging process; they've simply learned how to work with their skin, providing it with the nourishment and care it requires to flourish. There is no magic to it; it's all about knowledge and dedication.

Forget about the frustrating cycle of trial and error, or throwing money at expensive products that only make empty promises. We will explore the science behind skin health, busting myths and exposing the evidence-based practices that genuinely work. Consider this book to be your personal skincare advisor, guiding you on a journey of self-discovery and empowering beauty choices.

WHY TRUST US?

While you may not find a celebrity-like complexion on every member of the Ageless Revelations team (though some of us swear by the methods outlined here!), we've collectively dedicated years to research and experimentation. We understand the frustrations and disappointments you face in navigating the world of skincare.

Through relentless research, collaboration with leading dermatologists and aestheticians, and countless hours spent sifting through scientific studies, the Ageless Revelations team has assembled a wealth of information that can transform your approach to skincare.

Here are just a few of the shortcuts you'll discover with Ageless Revelations:

- **Science-based strategies:** Say goodbye to trendy and empty promises; this book uncovers the science behind effective skincare, giving you the knowledge to make informed decisions.
- **Tailored plans:** A one-size-fits-all approach is not the way to go here. Learn how to create a skincare regimen that caters to your unique skin type and concerns.
- **Time-efficient tips:** Find out about quick and efficient routines that fit seamlessly into your busy lifestyle, without compromising on results.
- **Professional advice:** Get access to the expertise of top dermatologists, aestheticians, and nutritionists, all summarized in an easy-to-follow guide.
- **Real-life success stories:** Explore the motivating stories of regular women (and men!) who have accomplished extraordinary outcomes using the techniques outlined in this book.

With this book, you'll not only achieve beautiful skin but also cultivate self-love and acceptance. You'll learn to appreciate your skin's unique journey and embrace its natural beauty at every stage of life. As part of the passionate Ageless Revelations team, dedicated to skin longevity, I've walked the path you're on and emerged with a roadmap to success. Trust me, with the knowledge and tools you'll gain from this book, your journey towards timeless beauty becomes a smooth, empowering adventure.

Are you ready to start his transformative journey? Turn the page, and let's begin!

CHAPTER 1
DECODING THE SCIENCE OF AGELESS SKIN

Think you know your skin? Take a moment to test your knowledge with this quick quiz:

1. The outermost layer of your skin is called the:

   - (a) Epidermis
   - (b) Dermis
   - (c) Hypodermis

2. As we age, our skin's natural ability to retain moisture:

   - (a) Increases
   - (b) Decreases
   - (c) Stays the same

3. Genetics play a significant role in determining:

   - (a) Skin type (oily, dry, etc.)
   - (b) Healing rate from sun damage
   - (c) Both (a) and (b)

Did you pick the correct answers? Were you confident in answering these questions? Probably not. Trust me, I didn't know either (back in my not-so-beautiful skin era). Let me ask you this, have you ever noticed a change in your skin over time? Perhaps you've observed a difference in its texture, tone, or elasticity. What do you think might have contributed to this change? For years to come, your skin can maintain its youthful glow and healthiness by learning all you can about its structure, how it ages naturally, and the role genetics plays.

THE MARVEL OF SKIN—ITS LAYERS AND FUNCTIONS

Did you know that your skin is the body's largest and most adaptable organ? It serves as a vigilant guard, a robust barrier against external factors, and a complex communication hub. Even though it's only two millimeters thick (equivalent to the width of two pennies), it flawlessly performs a wide array of functions that are essential for our well-being.

Firstly, our skin acts as a barrier, protecting us from UV rays, bacteria, and pollutants, like a suit of armor for our organs. Secondly, it helps the body keep its temperature stable by sweating and controlling blood flow. This is very important for proper working, and you can imagine tiny air conditioners and heaters working tirelessly beneath the surface.

In addition, feelings of touch, pressure, heat, and cold are sent to our brains through nerve endings that are embedded in our skin. Like a network of cell phone towers, these sensors are always sending information about our surroundings to our brain.

Last but not least, getting enough vitamin D—which your skin makes when exposed to sunshine—is essential for good health in general and for strong bones in particular. You might think of your skin's ability to absorb sunlight as a natural vitamin D factory, cranking out this essential ingredient.

It's truly amazing how our skin performs all these functions flawlessly. Layers of skin, each with its own job, are carefully arranged so that your skin can do these vital things. Now that we've established the basic structure of the skin, let's delve deeper into the fascinating world of each layer.

1. The Epidermis

Did you know that the epidermis is the first line of defense for your skin? It's pretty amazing! The epidermis is a self-renewing barrier that contains many important cell types, all of which are essential to its protective function. For instance, about 90% of the skin is made up of keratinocytes, which are constantly being made in the lower layers and slowly move to the top, where they exfoliate as dead skin cells. Keratin, a protein that gives the outer layer of skin its strength and waterproofing, is found in these cells.

Melanocytes are another important cell type found in the epidermis. These specialized cells make melanin, the pigment that gives skin and hair their color. Melanin can absorb the sun's ultraviolet (UV) rays and shield the skin's deeper layers from damage. That's pretty cool, right?

Finally, Langerhans cells are immune system's scouts that play a key role in detecting and eliminating harmful microbes and viruses that try to penetrate the skin's protective barrier. Without these cells, our skin would be more susceptible to infections and diseases.

2. The Dermis

Ever wonder what keeps your skin looking so good? It's not just a flat sheet! The dermis, the layer beneath the surface, is like a bustling city with two key districts. The top part, the papillary dermis, is a sensory haven. Think of it as a neighborhood with lots of cafés (blood vessels delivering nutrients) and parks (sensory receptors). It keeps the outer layer of skin, the epidermis, informed about what's going on (feeling touch, warmth) and gives it the fuel it needs to stay healthy.

Then, there's the reticular dermis, the city's strong underbelly. Here, collagen acts like steel beams in a building, giving your skin its strength and keeping wrinkles at bay. Unfortunately, collagen production slows down as we age, just like those weekend DIY projects start to pile up!

Elastin is another key player; it's like a network of rubber bands woven throughout the dermis. These fibers keep your skin elastic, allowing it to stretch and bounce back. But you guessed it, elastin production also dips as we get older, which is why things get a little less bouncy over time.

3. The Hypodermis

Don't underestimate the fluffy layer under your skin! The hypodermis, often demonized for holding onto fat, is actually a total party hero. Think of it as a super-insulated VIP lounge for your insides. That layer of fat keeps you warm in the winter and cool in the summer, acting like a built-in thermostat. Plus, it's a shock absorber, protecting your organs from bumps and bruises.

But fat isn't all about padding! Those fat cells are actually tiny energy tanks, ready to fuel your body whenever it needs a boost. They're like an internal gas station, keeping you going throughout the day. And let's not forget the aesthetics! The amount of fat in your hypodermis determines your curves and facial fullness. A well-padded hypodermis can keep you looking youthful and plump, while a depleted one might leave you looking a bit gaunt.

4. Appendages-Hair Follicles, Sweat Glands, and Sebaceous Glands

Skin isn't just a layered wonder, it's also home to some fascinating little party guests! Let's meet a few VIPs. First up, the hair follicles! These tiny pockets are the hair growth headquarters, where each strand starts its journey. But they're not loners—they have built-in sebaceous gland buddies. These little oil factories pump out sebum, a magic potion that keeps your hair and skin from becoming a dry, itchy mess.

Next, we have the sweat glands, scattered all over like a built-in sprinkler system. When things get heated (literally!), these guys release sweat, a watery layer that cools you down as it evaporates. Think of them as your personal AC unit, keeping you from overheating on the dance floor.

And don't forget the sebaceous glands again! These multitasking marvels, located near hair follicles, also produce sebum to keep your skin and hair nicely moisturized. But just like any good party, too much of a good thing can happen. Overactive sebaceous glands can lead to acne breakouts, so finding a balance is key!

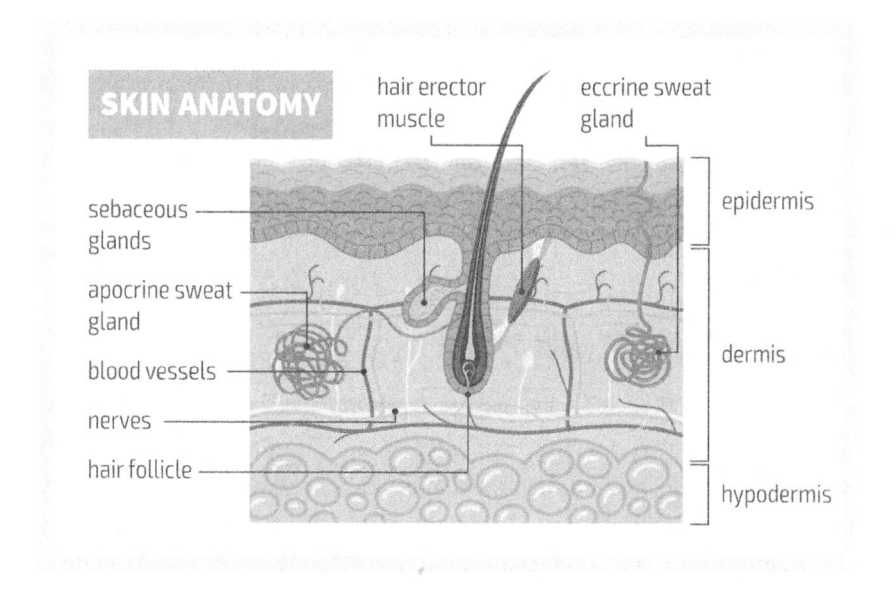

SKIN ANATOMY AND RECENT ADVANCEMENTS

Our skin is very remarkable, isn't it? But experts always try to find better ways to do things. Skin bioengineering is a novel and exciting area that can help with it. Can you picture yourself with lab-grown artificial skin? Isn't it incredibly futuristic?

This technology could be very helpful for people with burns, long-term scars, or even some skin diseases. They are basically making skin patches that will help people heal faster and leave less of a scar. Plus, they could use each person's own cells to make these patches fit perfectly, which would be great for lowering the risk of rejection.

Bioengineered skin could also be used to send medicine right to where it's needed, which is another intriguing idea. Think about it—targeted treatment with fewer side effects! That seems nice, doesn't it? Of course, this is all brand-new ground. It's not easy to make skin that is as complicated as ours, and it's even harder to make it cheap and easy for everyone to get. Aside from that, we need to think about things like ethics and make sure this technology is used in a good way.

However, researchers are making great progress! They are always learning how to do amazing things like heal and protect us from the outside world that our skin does naturally. Some people even think that this technology could one day be used to control body temperature, which would be crazy! Even though it's still early, skin technology could change the way we treat skin problems in big ways. It's like starting a new book in skin care, and I can't wait to see what comes next!

UNDERSTANDING HOW SKIN AGES

Aging, let's face it, it's like that pesky to-do list—it just keeps growing! But just like you can prioritize tasks, we can prioritize healthy skin habits to keep it glowing. Our skin, much like a beautiful garden, needs constant care to flourish as time goes by. Did you know wrinkles are the number one skin concern globally (Culliney, 2023). No wonder, those unwanted lines can be a real downer.

So, what's happening beneath the surface? Imagine your skin as a vibrant garden. Collagen and elastin are like the strong trellis supporting climbing flowers, keeping everything youthful and plump. Hyaluronic acid acts as the garden's watering system, ensuring all the plants stay hydrated and healthy. But as time marches on, the garden undergoes some changes.

As we age, collagen and elastin production naturally slows down. Picture the trellis getting a little weak and needing repairs. This loss of support can lead to wrinkles and sagging, just like wilting flowers.

Hyaluronic acid, our skin's water source, starts to dwindle. Think of the irrigation system leaking, leaving the plants thirsty. This dehydration causes dryness, fine lines, and a loss of that youthful glow.

Sun exposure is like pesky weeds in our garden. UV rays break down collagen and elastin, just like weeds stealing nutrients from the flowers. This speeds up aging and leads to sunspots, wrinkles, and uneven skin tone.

The Effects We See

As we age, our skin undergoes a series of internal changes that eventually become visible on the surface. The loss of collagen and elastin, the building blocks of youthful skin, take a major toll. This decline is like cracks appearing in the foundation of a city, leading to the formation of wrinkles and fine lines, especially noticeable around the eyes, lips, and forehead. Elasticity, which keeps our skin looking springy and youthful, also suffers when elastin production drops. Imagine once-tall buildings starting to tilt and lean— that's what happens to our jawline, neck, and jowls as they lose elasticity.

Hyaluronic acid, another key player in healthy skin, plays a crucial role in hydration. As hyaluronic acid levels decrease, the skin becomes dehydrated and loses its plumpness. This dehydration is like the city fountains running dry and parks withering away—the skin loses its youthful glow and becomes dull. Sun exposure adds another layer of complexity. Over time, the sun's harmful rays contribute to uneven skin tone, causing both hyperpigmentation (dark patches) and hypopigmentation (lighter patches). Imagine the city buildings getting faded and patchy over time due to bad weather—that's a similar effect the sun has on our skin.

It's important to remember that aging is a gradual process, and the pace at which these changes manifest varies from person to person. Genetics, lifestyle choices, and sun exposure all play a significant role in how our skin ages. The good news is that while we can't turn back time, we can significantly influence the rate of skin aging through the choices we make. By understanding what's happening beneath the surface, we can take charge and develop a skincare routine that combats the visible signs of aging.

THE CAUSES OF SKIN AGING

Let's face it, we all love the way our skin looks when we're young and glowing. But as time marches on, things start to change. Wrinkles pop up, that youthful bounce fades, and let's be honest, sunspots aren't exactly a welcome addition. But what exactly causes this to happen? Well, it's not just one thing to blame. It's actually a combination of two main factors: What's going on inside our bodies (intrinsic factors) and how we live our lives (extrinsic factors). Understanding these two sides of the coin is key to fighting back against skin aging.

The Inside Story

Our genes play a big role in how our skin ages. They kind of set the baseline for things like how fast our collagen production slows down and how susceptible we are to sun damage. We'll get more into the specifics of genes later, but for now, just know they have a say in the game.

On top of genes, other internal things can influence how our skin ages too. For example, as our hormone levels change, especially estrogen and testosterone, our skin can lose some of its firmness and elasticity. Think of it like a bouncy castle slowly losing air—that's kind of what happens!

There's also this thing called cellular senescence, which is a fancy way of saying our skin cells get tired over time and don't work quite as well. This can lead to slower skin renewal and less overall healthy-looking skin.

The Outside World

Our daily lives play a surprising role in how our skin ages! Sun exposure is a big villain in this story. Those UV rays act like tiny thieves, stealing your youthful glow and leading to wrinkles, fine lines, and uneven skin tone. That's why sunscreen is your BFF! Smoking is another culprit—it cuts off the blood flow to your skin, starving it of the nutrients and oxygen it needs to stay healthy. This translates to premature wrinkles and a dull complexion—not exactly the look we're going for.

What you eat matters too! Skimping on vitamins, minerals, and antioxidants can accelerate skin aging. Think of these nutrients as tiny warriors fighting free radicals that damage your skin and keeping it healthy. Feeling stressed all the time can also wreak havoc. It can make your skin inflamed, weaken its natural barrier, and amplify all those other signs of aging.

Here's a cool fact: There's a whole world of bacteria living on your skin, called the skin microbiome! Scientists are still figuring things out, but it seems these tiny tenants might play a role in how your skin ages. Who knows, maybe this research will lead to new ways to keep our skin looking youthful!

ROLE OF GENES IN SKIN AGING

We've been talking about the double whammy of skin aging: internal factors, like collagen loss, and external ones, like sun damage. But there's another player in the game—your genes! Think of them as a complex instruction manual that dictates things like how thick your skin is naturally, how quickly it heals itself, and even how sensitive it is to the sun. These instructions vary a lot from person to person, and that can influence how quickly your skin shows signs of aging.

Now, here's the good news: Genes aren't the whole story. Even if you got dealt a hand with some not-so-great skin aging instructions, there's still a lot you can do! Here's why:

First, genes don't always shout at full volume. Lifestyle choices can actually influence how your genes are expressed. For example, if you have a genetic tendency to be more susceptible to sun damage, a healthy diet packed with antioxidants can help fight back.

Second, while you can't rewrite your genetic code, you can focus on the things you can control. Sun protection, healthy habits, and a good skincare routine can all significantly impact how your skin ages, regardless of what your genes say. So, the power to keep your skin looking great is still very much in your hands!

The Rate of Aging

Genes turn out to be like a personal roadmap for how our skin ages! They influence things like the speed at which our collagen production naturally slows down (think of collagen as the building blocks that keep your skin firm and bouncy). Genes with names like COL1A1 and COL3A1 might sound like a mouthful, but they basically determine how quickly those building blocks start to disappear.

Another way genes play a role is in skin repair. Imagine your skin is a battlefield against sun damage—some genes are like skilled repair crews, patching things up quickly. Others, well, maybe not so much. This can affect how many wrinkles and fine lines show up over time. Genes can even influence how well wounds heal and scar.

Genetic Predispositions and Common Skin Conditions

Genes can also be like tiny booby traps when it comes to skin! Some genes can make you more prone to certain skin conditions that can speed up the aging process. Acne, for example, is a battle where genes can ramp up oil production and inflammation, both of which lead to those pesky breakouts (thanks to research by Sutaria and Schlessinger in 2019) (Sutaria & Schlessinger, 2019). Eczema, that itchy, irritated skin condition, also has a strong genetic link. It seems variations in genes that control your skin's barrier function can play a role. Psoriasis, another chronic skin issue, has a complex genetic component too. Certain genes can make you more likely to develop it.

But here's the good news: Even if you have a family history of these conditions, it's not all doom and gloom! By knowing your predispositions, you can be proactive. Keeping up with a healthy diet, regular exercise, and a fantastic skincare routine can all help you fight back. Who knows? You might even end up looking younger than your actual age by taking charge of your skin's health!

SUMMARY

- The three layers of skin—the epidermis (the outer layer), the dermis (the middle layer), and the hypodermis (the bottom layer)—make it the biggest and most intricate organ in the body.
- Both internal (genes, hormones) and environmental (sun exposure, smoking, food) factors contribute to skin aging.
- Common signs of aging skin include wrinkles, dryness, and uneven skin tone.
- While genetics play a role in how quickly your skin ages, you can significantly influence this process through healthy lifestyle choices and a good skincare routine.
- Taking charge of your skin health can help you maintain a youthful appearance for longer.

SEGUE

So, we just peeled back the layers (literally) on our amazing skin. We saw it's not just a pretty face, but a super-powered shield, temperature regulator, and even a tiny vitamin factory! But, hey, even superheroes get a few wrinkles after a while, right? Our skin shows some wear and tear as we age, but the good news is we can slow that process down! By understanding what makes skin age and taking care of it, we can keep that youthful glow going strong.

Traditionally, skincare routines focus on what we put on our face. But what about what goes *in* our bodies? Next chapter, we'll ditch the wrinkles and dryness for good by focusing on nourishing your skin from the inside out! We'll explore how food, drinks, and even your sleep makes a big difference in how your skin looks and feels. Get ready to learn how to give your skin the ultimate internal glow-up!

CHAPTER 2
NOURISHING YOUR SKIN FROM WITHIN

Have you ever seen someone who looks like they bottled the fountain of youth? That's Chuando Tan in a nutshell. This Singaporean model and photographer is going to hit 60 this year, but trust me, you'd never guess it by looking at his impossibly youthful face and ripped physique. He's basically a walking advertisement for defying Father Time!

Therefore, how does Chuando do it? The answer, my dear, is an intriguing story. While his secret sauce might not be a one-size-fits-all deal (because, let's face it, our skin is as unique as our fingerprints), Chuando's journey to agelessness offers some serious clues. We're talking about the power of good choices, from the food he eats to how he cares for his skin.

Prepare to say goodbye to the time machine because, in this chapter, we're about to uncover the secret behind Chuando's everlasting youthfulness. We will explore the secrets of skin-loving nutrients, the significance of maintaining proper hydration (imagine an inner and outward glow!), and the unexpected influence of your diet. Stay tuned because I'm about to spill the tea on the meaning of everlasting beauty, and you're going to be quite amazed!

A DEEP DIVE INTO SKIN-FRIENDLY NUTRIENTS

Looking for the perfect skin care product can be a never-ending search. However, the key to achieving radiant skin might be closer than you think—on your dinner plate. Our skin requires nourishment, just like any other living organ. Think of it like a garden: Without the right nutrients, it won't flourish. The same goes for our skin, which needs specific vitamins, minerals, and healthy fats to maintain its health, suppleness, and inner glow.

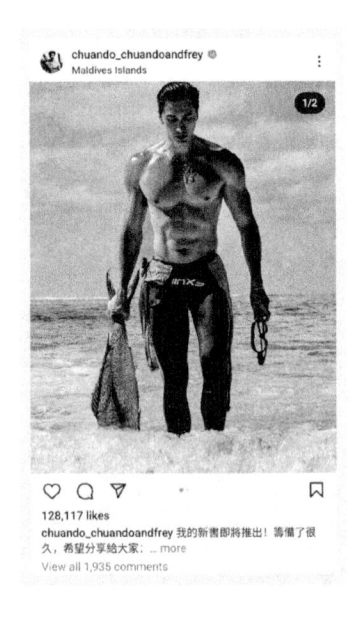

While topical treatments can offer temporary benefits, long-lasting results come from taking care of our skin from the inside out. Various studies published in the National Institutes of Health have shown a clear link between our dietary choices and the condition of our skin (Sharma et al., 2024). These studies observed that people who consume a diet rich in specific nutrients experienced improvements in skin hydration, elasticity, and even a reduction in wrinkles. So, what are these magical ingredients that can boost our skin? Let's explore!

Vitamin A: The Collagen Champion

Concerning skin health, vitamin A is a miracle. It is an essential regulator of cell proliferation and differentiation, and it is involved in the synthesis of collagen, the structural protein that maintains the plump appearance of skin. Getting enough vitamin A can help with skin suppleness, wrinkles, and acne. Just so you know, sweet potatoes are packed with vitamin A. Also, they are an essential part of Chuando Tan's diet, which helps him maintain his youthful appearance.

Food sources: sweet potatoes, carrots, pumpkin, kale, spinach, cantaloupe, eggs, and full-fat dairy products.

Vitamin C: The Antioxidant Avenger

Our skin is constantly bombarded by free radicals—unstable molecules generated by sun exposure, pollution, and even normal cellular processes. Cell damage caused by these free radicals causes the skin to look older than it actually is, with wrinkles and a lackluster general tone. Vitamin C comes to the rescue as a potent antioxidant, neutralizing free radicals before they can wreak havoc. Research suggests that consuming sufficient vitamin C can improve skin texture, reduce wrinkles, and even offer some protection against sun damage.

Food sources: citrus fruits (oranges, grapefruits, lemons), bell peppers, kiwis, broccoli, strawberries, and guava.

Vitamin D: The Sunshine Ally

Although the majority of us link vitamin D with strong bones, it turns out that this vitamin from the sun also has an important role in maintaining healthy skin. Skin problems like eczema and atopic dermatitis might come up for not getting enough vitamin D. Vitamin D may help the skin's barrier function and maybe even prevent it from UV damage.

Food sources: fatty fish (salmon, tuna, sardines), egg yolks, fortified milk and cereals, mushrooms (exposed to sunlight). However, getting enough vitamin D from food alone can be challenging. Consider discussing supplementation with your doctor.

Vitamin E: The Anti-Inflammatory Champion

Vitamin E joins the fight for healthy skin as another powerful antioxidant. It not only shields your skin from sun damage but also helps reduce inflammation, which can manifest as redness, irritation, and even acne. Vitamin E can hydrate the skin better and maybe lessen the look of wrinkles.

Food sources: almonds, avocados, sunflower seeds, olive oil, spinach, and kiwi.

Vitamin K: The Healing Hero

The proper functioning of the skin depends on vitamin K's ability to clot blood and repair wounds. Vitamin K's potential topical advantages are still under study, but it does help diminish the look of fine lines and wrinkles, such as spider veins and dark circles under the eyes.

Food sources: broccoli, Brussels sprouts, asparagus, kale, spinach, collard greens, and fermented foods such as natto.

Omega-3 Fatty Acids: The Moisture Marvels

Imagine your skin as a tightly woven net, with each strand representing a healthy fat molecule. Omega-3 fatty acids, particularly those found in oily fish, form the foundation of your skin's natural moisture barrier. This barrier acts like a shield, keeping essential moisture locked in and preventing environmental aggressors from entering. When your skin lacks sufficient omega-3s, the moisture barrier weakens, leading to dryness, flakiness, and even irritation.

Food sources: fatty fish (salmon, tuna, sardines, mackerel), flaxseeds, chia seeds, walnuts, and eggs.

ESSENTIAL MINERALS

While vitamins often steal the spotlight when it comes to skin health, essential minerals play an equally crucial role. These powerhouse ingredients act behind the scenes, orchestrating various functions that keep your skin healthy, resilient, and radiant. Let's delve into three essential minerals—zinc, selenium, and copper—and explore how they contribute to a healthy complexion:

Zinc: The Healing Hero

Zinc is a multitasking mineral with a profound impact on skin health. One of its most important functions is regulating oil production in the skin. Excessive oil production can clog pores and lead to breakouts, but zinc helps keep things balanced, promoting a clearer complexion. Studies have shown that zinc supplementation can be beneficial in managing acne, particularly inflammatory acne (Cherney, 2018).

Zinc is important for skin health for reasons beyond only controlling oil production, it speeds wound healing and promotes cell regeneration. Zinc also has antioxidant qualities that are great for warding off free radical damage, which is a leading cause of skin aging.

Food sources: oysters, lean beef, chicken, chickpeas, lentils, pumpkin seeds, cashews, and dark chocolate (cocoa content 70% or higher).

Selenium: The Antioxidant Ally

The battle against free radicals also includes selenium, another potent antioxidant. In a complementary fashion with vitamin E, it protects the skin from the sun's rays, preventing premature aging, hyperpigmentation, and cancer. Those who consume enough selenium have fewer wrinkles and fine lines, giving the impression that they are younger than they actually are (Michalak et al., 2021). Another one of Chuando Tan's secrets!

Food sources: Brazil nuts (in moderation due to high selenium content), seafood (tuna, salmon, sardines), eggs, chicken, whole grains (brown rice, quinoa), and mushrooms.

Copper: The Collagen Powerhouse

Copper, sometimes called the "beauty mineral," is essential for the body to make collagen. Loss of collagen production is a normal consequence of aging, which causes skin to become less supple and wrinkles to appear. On top of that, copper has anti-inflammatory qualities that can ease red, inflamed skin and speed up the healing process.

Food sources: oysters, liver (consume in moderation), shiitake mushrooms, sesame seeds, cashews, avocados, and dark chocolate (cocoa content 70% or higher).

The best way to make sure you're getting enough of these minerals is to eat a balanced diet. Supplements may be helpful in certain situations, but before starting any new supplement regimen, it's wise to talk to your doctor.

The Synergy of Skin Health

Both the unique properties and the synergistic effects of these vital minerals are what make them so appealing. A potent symphony of zinc, selenium, copper, and the vitamins we just covered helps maintain healthy skin. You can give your skin the nutrients it needs to flourish by eating a varied diet that is high in these nutrients.

ANTIOXIDANTS VS FREE RADICALS

Imagine millions of tiny, unstable molecules constantly bombarding your skin, like an army of microscopic vandals. The skin's health and attractiveness are seriously jeopardized by these free radicals. Because they lack an electron pair, free radicals are very reactive oxygen molecules that have gone rogue. In their pursuit of stability, they oxidize healthy skin cells to obtain electrons. This loss of cells throws off the delicate balance inside your skin cells, which causes a condition called oxidative stress.

Think of your skin cells as meticulously organized factories. Free radicals are like rogue workers who barge in and wreak havoc. They damage the machinery (cellular structures) and disrupt production (healthy skin components). This oxidative stress manifests in a number of ways that accelerate the aging process of your skin.

Oxidative stress is basically a war happening right inside your skin cells! This war speeds up how fast your skin ages and shows itself in a few not-so-fun ways. First, free radicals damage collagen and elastin, those amazing proteins that keep your skin looking plump and bouncy. This damage leads to wrinkles and fine lines. Moreover, your skin loses its elasticity, making it look saggy. To make matters worse, free radicals can mess with melanin, your skin's pigment. This can lead to uneven skin tone and dark spots. Not exactly the youthful glow we're all after!

Does all of that make you worried? Don't be. Antioxidants are here to protect you from these harmful free radicals! These powerful molecules act as nature's defense system, neutralizing free radicals before they can damage your skin cells. Think of them as tiny shields, absorbing the extra electron from free radicals and rendering them harmless, like valiant knights deflecting the attacks of a ferocious dragon.

We've already explored the antioxidant power of several essential vitamins such as vitamin C, E, and K. Let's take a look at other antioxidant army that can help you revitalize your skin.

Expanding the Antioxidant Army

The fight against free radicals doesn't stop there. Let's introduce some additional antioxidant all-stars:

Coenzyme Q10 (CoQ10)

The body's production of this antioxidant naturally decreases as we get older. Aside from potentially reducing the visibility of wrinkles, its primary function is to shield skin cells from harm. You can get your daily dose of CoQ10 from fatty fish, moderately consumed organ meats, and a few nuts and seeds.

Green Tea

Loaded with polyphenols, a class of powerful antioxidants, green tea helps combat free radical damage and may offer some protection against sun damage. Green tea is a fantastic source of antioxidants, and rumor has it, Chuando Tan starts his day with a steaming cup! Enjoy green tea hot or iced, or explore skincare products containing green tea extract.

Lycopene

People who eat tomatoes and other red foods may be less likely to get sunburn, and their skin may stay healthy from sun damage (Story et al., 2010). In such case, savor those tomato-based summer salads and dishes!

Resveratrol

Found in red grapes, red wine (consumed in moderation), and peanuts, resveratrol is another antioxidant warrior with potential benefits for skin health. Studies suggest it may help protect against sun damage and improve skin elasticity (News in Health, 2017).

Flavonoids

This diverse group of antioxidants found in fruits, vegetables, and dark chocolate (cocoa content 70% or higher) offer a variety of skin benefits. They can help reduce inflammation, protect against sun damage, and even promote collagen production.

You can help your skin fight free radicals and look younger by eating foods rich in antioxidants and using skincare products that include these nutrients. A robust antioxidant defense system begins with a balanced diet that is high in produce, whole grains, protein, and healthy fats.

HYDRATION AND SKIN ELASTICITY

Remember that time you spent all summer trying that fad mask everyone was talking about? Yeah, me too! We've all been there, searching for magic bullets. But the truth is, achieving healthy skin is more about consistent habits than quick fixes. Your skin is just like the coolest trampoline ever—the kind that lets you jump super high and always bounces you right back.

That's what skin elasticity is all about—it's how your skin stretches and snaps back into place, keeping it looking youthful. Collagen, a fancy word for a special protein, acts like the trampoline's frame, giving your skin that bounce. But just like a dusty old trampoline loses its fun factor, dehydrated skin gets all sad and saggy, leading to wrinkles, fine lines, and that *blah* complexion.

Here's where water comes in! Drinking enough H_2O is key to keeping your skin elastic. Think of your skin cells as juicy grapes. When they're well-hydrated, they stay plump and contribute to that smooth, glowy look we all love. But when they're dehydrated, they shrivel up like raisins, making your skin lose its bounce and more prone to wrinkles. Science even backs this up—studies show that drinking more water can improve your skin's hydration, elasticity, and overall awesomeness (Manalo, n.d.). While Chuando Tan might have a team of skincare experts, the secret weapon behind his youthful glow might be a simple one—staying hydrated! He reportedly carries a reusable water bottle everywhere he goes.

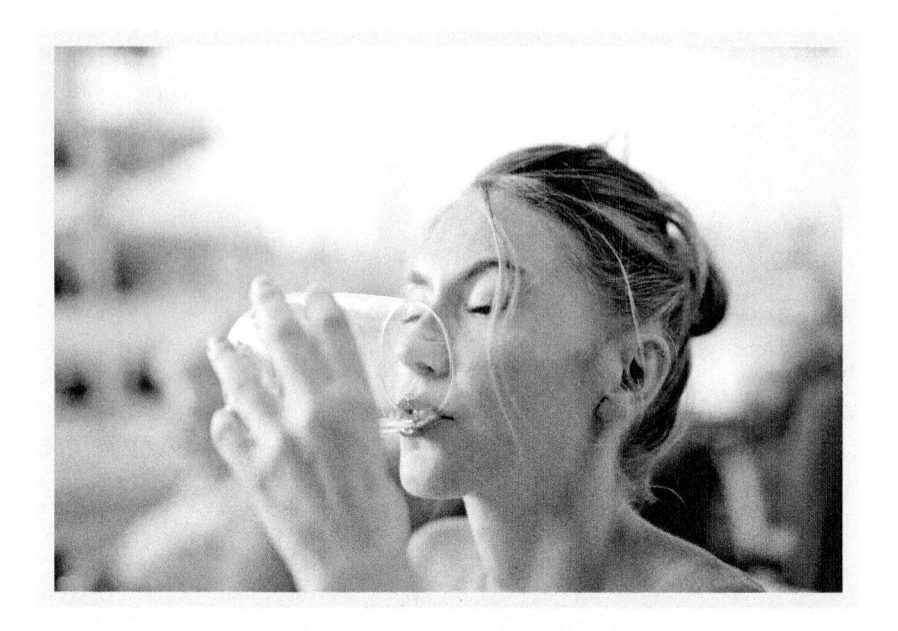

Dehydration vs Dry Skin

Ever wonder why your skin sometimes feels like a dried-up apple core, even though you use a moisturizer religiously? That might be a sign of dehydration, not dryness! It's like confusing being thirsty with having a leaky faucet. Dry skin is a skin type—it produces less oil naturally, making it feel rough and flaky. Dehydration, on the other hand, can happen to any skin type, even oily skin. It simply means your skin cells are lacking water, like a deflated pool float. So, how can you tell the difference between a dehydrated and dry skin? Here are some clues:

Dehydrated Skin:

- fine lines and wrinkles more prominent
- skin tight and uncomfortable
- dullness and lack of radiance
- dark circles under the eyes
- flaky patches (not always present)

Dry Skin:

- rough and scaly texture
- flaky patches
- increased sensitivity
- itching or irritation
- less visible pores

The Pinch Test

While the "pinch test" isn't a guaranteed way to diagnose dehydration, it can be a fun experiment. Pinch the skin on the back of your hand and hold for a few seconds. If it snaps back quickly, you're probably well-hydrated. But if it takes a while to bounce back, it could be a sign of dehydration. This isn't a foolproof method, so consulting a dermatologist is always a good idea for personalized advice.

Hydration Hacks for Happy Skin

Remember that bouncy trampoline we discussed before, symbolizing your skin's elasticity? Well, proper hydration acts like a constant stream of water, keeping it inflated and functioning perfectly. To achieve this, here are some fun and effective ways to keep your skin cells plump and your complexion glowing!

First things first—start your day hydrated! Just like your car needs gas for a smooth ride, your body needs water to function at its best. Aim for a glass of water as soon as you wake up, which will jumpstart your hydration and set the tone for a healthy day. Consider keeping a reusable water bottle by your bedside as a friendly reminder.

Next, pay attention to your physical sensations, not merely your taste buds. You should not wait until you are extremely thirsty before grabbing a bottle of water. Your body is trying to tell you, "Hey, I'm getting low on water!" when it feels thirsty. Even if you're not really thirsty, make it a habit to drink water throughout the day.

Feeling a little adventurous? Spice up your water game! While plain water is great, adding a little taste can encourage you to drink more. For an enjoyable variation, try slicing some cucumber, lemon, or berries and adding them to your water.

Here's a fun fact: You can actually eat your water! Many fruits and vegetables are loaded with water, making them a delicious way to hydrate. A diet rich in juicy fruits and vegetables, such as watermelon, cucumber, spinach, and strawberries, can do wonders for your skin.

Finally, tech can be your friend! If you want to keep tabs on how much water you drink each day, there are lots of applications for that. These apps can track your activity level and tailor your daily goals to suit your needs, including sending you reminders to drink. Therefore, make use of technology and watch your skin thrive!

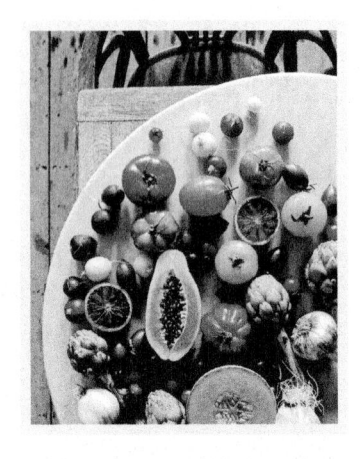

Beyond the Basics

Even though the previous tips are hydration rockstars, here are some extra moves to consider for an all-star hydration game plan:

First up, beat the heat! Hot weather sucks the moisture right out of you. When it's scorching outside, do your best to stay cool and avoid super intense workouts. Skincare can also be your hydration hero, but we'll save that deep dive for later. For now, know that certain lotions and creams can help lock moisture into your skin.

Speaking of hot water, those long steamy showers might feel amazing, but they can actually strip your skin's natural oils. Opt for lukewarm showers and keep them on the shorter side. Want to pamper yourself with a purpose? Face masks are a fun way to do it, and some can give your skin an extra hydration boost. Look for masks labeled "hydrating" or "moisturizing."

Here's a tech tip: Humidifiers add moisture to the air, which can be a lifesaver in dry climates or winter. This can help prevent your skin from drying out. And lastly, be mindful of your caffeine intake. While coffee and tea are great, they can dehydrate you. Balance out your caffeine with plenty of water throughout the day.

THE ANTI-INFLAMMATORY DIET FOR GLOWING SKIN

You wake up to a usual morning, walk towards the bathroom to freshen up and start your day when suddenly you look in the mirror and go, "Ew! When did that pop up? And out of all days, it had to be TODAY?" Well, that day was supposed to be flawless because you were supposed to nail that presentation, or visit an important person, or post your most-awaited video on Instagram. But those painful bumps ruined the day, and now you're looking for quick fixes.

That, my dear, is your skin freaking out after a weekend of greasy takeout and sugary treats. It's not just your imagination. Certain foods can trigger inflammation in your body, leading to redness, irritation, and unwelcome visitors like acne and eczema. However, there's a delicious solution: the anti-inflammatory diet! Chuando Tan is a big believer in a balanced diet, and that includes plenty of anti-inflammatory foods like fatty fish and green vegetables. Perhaps that's part of the reason his skin looks so calm and clear!

Think of your skin as a battlefield. Inflammatory triggers act like enemy soldiers, causing irritation and breakouts. An anti-inflammatory diet equips your body with powerful weapons—delicious, nutritious foods—to fight back and keep your skin calm and clear. Here's how this approach works:

The Inflammation Lowdown

Imagine your skin freaking out like a fire alarm going off for no reason! That's kind of what happens with inflammation. Your body's defense system, normally awesome at fighting off invaders, gets a little confused and goes into overdrive. This can happen for a bunch of reasons, like too much sun, harsh skincare products that irritate your skin, stress (hello, breakouts!), and even what you eat. That's right, food can be a major player in skin health. By loading up on anti-inflammatory foods, you can help your body calm down and give you that glowing, balanced complexion you deserve.

Therefore, here's your secret weapon against grumpy, inflamed skin: food! We're talking about a delicious way to fight back. First up, gotta talk about fatty fish like salmon, sardines, and mackerel. These guys are loaded with omega-3 fatty acids, which are basically nature's firefighters, taming inflammation all over your body, including your skin.

Next, let's get colorful! Fruits and veggies are like anti-inflammatory superheroes. Think berries, leafy greens, tomatoes, and bell peppers. They're packed with antioxidants and phytonutrients that fight off free radicals, those sneaky things that can cause inflammation. Olive oil also joins the party. This heart-healthy oil is rich in oleocanthal, a word that might be a tongue twister, but trust me, it's a powerful anti-inflammatory champ. Drizzle it on salads or use it for cooking—yum!

Tomatoes deserve a shoutout too. That red color? It comes from lycopene, an antioxidant that helps keep your skin calm. Don't forget about nuts and seeds! Almonds, walnuts, flaxseeds, and chia seeds are all superstars when it comes to omega-3s and fiber, both essential for keeping your skin healthy and happy. And last but not least, green tea! This drink is packed with polyphenols, which are basically antioxidants on steroids, helping to fight inflammation.

So, by making these superstars a regular part of your diet, you can help reduce skin inflammation and say hello to a calmer, clearer complexion. Now that's what I call a delicious victory!

The Mediterranean Magic

The Mediterranean diet deserves a special shout-out in the fight against inflammation. This dietary pattern emphasizes:

- whole grains
- fruits and vegetables
- fish and seafood
- healthy fats
- limited red meat and dairy

Many anti-inflammatory foods in this eating pattern may help with skin problems like acne and psoriasis. It's a tasty and effective way to reduce inflammation and get beautiful skin.

Foods that Fuel Inflammation

You've been loading your plate with anti-inflammatory superstars, which is awesome! But remember, knowledge is power, especially when it comes to fighting inflammation. Here's the thing: Some foods can actually trigger flare-ups. Let's break it down.

First on the hit list: processed food foes. These pre-packaged snacks and meals are loaded with refined sugars, unhealthy fats, and artificial ingredients—all inflammation instigators. So, ditch the processed stuff and embrace whole foods—your body will thank you for it!

Next up, the sugar showdown. Sugar crashes aren't the only battle you're facing. Excessive sugar intake can actually trigger inflammation throughout your body. Instead, swap out refined sugars for natural sweeteners or grab some fruit to satisfy your sweet tooth.

Red meat isn't completely off-limits, but think of it as a special occasion treat. Studies suggest it can ramp up inflammation. If you do have it, choose lean cuts. And remember, there are other protein sources that are inflammation fighters, like fish and beans, so focus on those instead.

Refined carbohydrates are another culprit. We're talking white bread, pastries, and sugary cereals. These guys can cause spikes in your blood sugar, which can contribute to inflammation. Whole grains are your new best friend here.

Lastly, the dairy dilemma (for some). If you have a hunch that dairy might be a trigger for your skin woes, try limiting it or cutting it out completely for a while. See if your skin clears up! Everyone's body reacts differently, so listen to yours and experiment with different foods to see what makes your skin feel fantastic. Remember, you're the master chef of your own health journey!

KICKSTART YOUR GLOW: A SAMPLE ANTI-INFLAMMATORY MEAL PLAN

Here's a delicious one-day sample meal plan featuring anti-inflammatory ingredients to keep your skin happy and healthy:

Meal	Dish	Recipe	Highlights
Breakfast	Antioxidant smoothie	Blend together 1 cup Greek yogurt, 1 cup frozen mixed berries (like raspberries, blueberries, and strawberries), ½ banana, a handful of spinach, and a splash of almond milk for a creamy and refreshing start to your day.	This smoothie is packed with antioxidants from the berries and spinach, and the Greek yogurt provides protein for sustained energy.
Lunch	Salmon nicoise salad	1. Grill or bake a salmon fillet (around 4-6 oz) seasoned with salt, pepper, and your favorite herbs (like lemon pepper or dill). 2. While the salmon cooks, prepare a bed of mixed greens (such as romaine, arugula, or a mix). Top with chopped tomatoes, red onion, and black olives.	This salad offers a satisfying combination of protein (from the salmon), healthy fats (from the olive oil), and vitamins (from the vegetables).

		3. Once cooked, flake the salmon and arrange it over the salad. 4. Drizzle with a light lemon vinaigrette (made with olive oil, lemon juice, salt, and pepper).	
Snack	Trail mix with a twist	Combine ½ cup of a mixture of almonds, walnuts, and dried cranberries.	This mix provides healthy fats (from the nuts), fiber (from the almonds and walnuts), and a touch of sweetness and antioxidants (from the cranberries). Feel free to adjust the nut and dried fruit combination based on your preferences.
Dinner	One-pan chicken with roasted vegetables	1. Preheat oven to 400°F (200°C). 2. Season 2 boneless, skinless chicken breasts with herbs like rosemary, thyme, salt, and pepper. 3. In a bowl, combine olive oil, salt, and pepper with chopped vegetables. This might include 1 cup of broccoli florets, 1 cup of cherry tomatoes, and 1 cup of red bell pepper slices. 4. Arrange the chicken breasts and vegetables on a baking sheet. 5. Roast in the oven for 20 to 25 minutes, or until chicken is fully cooked and veggies are soft and crunchy.	The chicken gives this dish lean protein, the olive oil good fats, and the veggies are a great source of vitamins and antioxidants. With this one-pan method, cleaning up is a breeze!

Bonus tip: Throughout the day, aim to drink plenty of water to stay hydrated and support your skin's health.

Remember, this is just a sample plan. Feel free to explore different anti-inflammatory recipes and ingredients to create a meal plan that suits your taste and preferences!

SUMMARY

This chapter has taught us that

- specific vitamins and minerals like vitamin A, C, E, D, K, omega-3s, zinc, selenium, and copper play a crucial role in skin health.
- antioxidants like CoQ10, green tea, lycopene, resveratrol, and flavonoids fight free radicals that damage skin cells.
- proper hydration is essential for maintaining skin elasticity. Dehydrated skin looks dull and wrinkled.
- an anti-inflammatory diet rich in fatty fish, fruits, vegetables, olive oil, nuts, seeds, and green tea can promote clear and calm skin.
- limit processed foods, sugar, red meat, refined carbohydrates, and dairy (for some) as they can trigger inflammation.

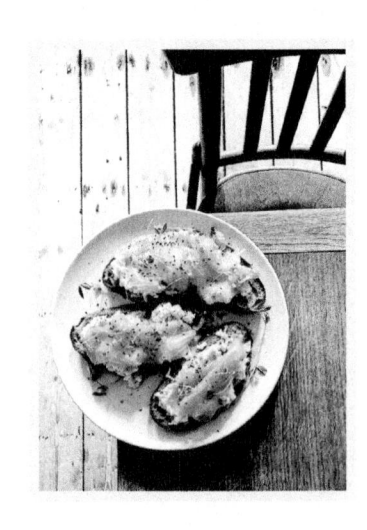

SEGUE

What are the takeaways from the science and story of Chuando Tan? If you want your skin to look healthy and radiant, you need to take care of your mental and emotional health first. Taking care of your skin and preserving its youthful shine is as easy as adopting certain changes to your diet.

Now, we'll examine the ways in which your way of living ruins your skin's radiant party. We're going to lay out the cold, hard facts regarding the ways in which things like smoking and alcohol harm the skin. Rest assured, we have solutions to address these issues! Turn the page and keep reading!

CHAPTER 3
LIFESTYLE FACTORS AND SKIN AGING

Have you ever scrolled through social media, mesmerized by celebrities with seemingly ageless complexions? You peek at your own reflection and wonder—what's their secret? Is it a team of dermatologists and a beauty cabinet overflowing with exotic potions? Perhaps. But the truth is, there's more to radiant skin than just the products you slather on.

Consider Julia as an example. She has an overflowing beauty cabinet and follows a 10-step skincare routine religiously. However, she might be missing a crucial ingredient—a lifestyle that complements her meticulous skincare efforts. Certain unhealthy habits, such as late-night Netflix binges that turn into early mornings, constant work deadlines, and regular indulgences in cigarettes and cocktails, can harm the health of her skin, even though they may seem unrelated.

This chapter is your key to the world where your lifestyle choices and your skin have a conversation. So, if you've ever felt like your skincare routine is fighting a losing battle, consider this your declaration of independence! This chapter is your guide to unlocking the secrets of glowing skin from the inside out. Get ready to transform your lifestyle and witness the transformation of your skin!

HOW SMOKING STEALS YOUR SKIN'S GLOW

Did you know that smoking not only messes up your health but also wreaks havoc on your skin? Yep, those sticks of cigarettes contain over 4,000 harmful chemicals that can damage your skin at a cellular level (Canadian Lung Association, 2016). Smoking fast-forwards the breakdown of collagen and elastin, which are the building blocks of firm, plump skin. So, if you want to avoid wrinkles, sagging, and unwanted fine lines or crow's feet, you might want to put that cigarette down.

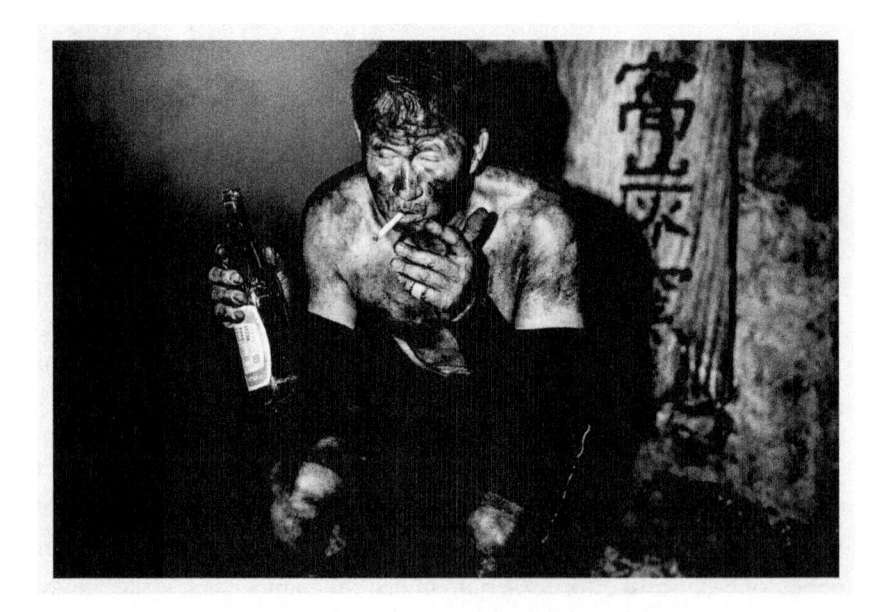

Plus, the facial expressions smokers make while puffing, such as pursed lips and squinting eyes, can deepen wrinkles over time. How's that for a reason to quit smoking? Also, smoking constricts blood vessels, which limits the flow of oxygen and nutrients to your skin cells. So, not only does your skin look dull and lifeless, but it also becomes more prone to breakouts, irritation, and even minor cuts or scrapes.

Lastly, smoking can also cause hyperpigmentation (dark spots) and uneven skin tone. So, instead of a healthy, even glow, you might end up with blotchy patches. Not cool, right? So, if you're looking to maintain your youthful and healthy skin, ditching that smoking habit would be a great start. Trust me, your skin (and your body) will thank you for it!

Quitting and Seeing the Results

Alright, you've quit smoking, high five! Now, get ready for some amazing things to happen to your skin. First up, improved blood flow! Within weeks of quitting, you might notice a rosy flush returning to your face. That's because blood is finally flowing freely again, delivering oxygen and nutrients straight to your skin cells. Think of it as a VIP pass to the nourishment station, keeping your skin healthy and radiant.

Next, your body's natural healing abilities get a major boost. This means breakouts will clear up faster, and any wounds you have will heal more quickly. So, goodbye stubborn pimples and hello smoother, clearer skin! Over time, with consistent smoke-free living, you might even see a more even skin tone. That pesky hyperpigmentation? It could start to fade away, revealing a brighter, more radiant complexion.

And here's the cherry on top: Quitting smoking can slow down future collagen breakdown. Collagen is the key player that keeps your skin plump and youthful. By slowing down the breakdown, you might see a reduction in the appearance of wrinkles. So, quitting not only helps your health but also helps you age gracefully—win-win!

Real People, Real Skin Transformations

Let's look at some real stories from people who experienced a skin glow-up after ditching cigarettes from sources such as Reddit, PatientsLikeMe, and QuitSure:

From Reddit—The HappyNonSmoker

"I smoked for 15 years and my skin was constantly dull and looked older than my age. I finally quit 6 months ago, and the biggest difference I've noticed is in my skin. It's so much brighter and healthier-looking now! I can't believe the difference quitting has made" (antigoneelectra, 2021).

PatientsLikeMe—The SmokesFreeSince30

"For years, I battled persistent acne and uneven skin tone. I tried every cream and potion under the sun, but nothing worked. Finally, I decided to quit smoking. It wasn't easy, but after a few months, I started to see a change. My breakouts became less frequent, and my skin tone began to even out. Now, a year smoke-free, my skin is clearer and brighter than it's ever been. Quitting smoking was the best decision I've ever made for my health and my skin!" (Mary, 2023).

QuitSure—Review on a Smoking Cessation App

"I never realized how much smoking was affecting my skin until I quit. I had these deep wrinkles around my eyes and mouth that seemed to appear overnight. After quitting with QuitSure's help, I noticed my skin started to look smoother and healthier. The wrinkles are still there, but they're not as deep anymore. Plus, my skin has a natural glow that I haven't seen in years. I feel so much better about myself now, both inside and out!"

These are just a few examples, and everyone's journey is unique. But the message is clear: Quitting smoking can have a positive impact on your skin. It's an investment in your overall health and well-being, and the results can be truly rewarding.

ALCOHOL—DEHYDRATION PARTY CRASHER FOR YOUR SKIN!

Ever notice your skin looking dull and feeling tight after a night of drinks? It's not just a hangover feeling! Alcohol can actually wreak havoc on your complexion. Here's the lowdown on how excessive boozing can impact your skin's health.

First up, dehydration disaster. Your skin needs air and water to stay plump and happy. Alcohol hogs all the water, leaving your skin dehydrated and deflated. Studies like one published in the Journal of the American Academy of Dermatology (think fancy science talk for skin doctors!) even show how alcohol disrupts your skin's natural ability to retain moisture (Li et al., 2017). This translates to dullness, flakiness, and irritation—not exactly the post-party glow you were hoping for!

Also, being dehydrated makes wrinkles and fine lines show up faster. Alcohol can make you go to the bathroom more often, which can dry out your skin. Science backs this up! The International Journal of Cancer published a study that found a link between heavy drinking and skin that ages faster than it should (Yahya Mahamat-Saleh et al., 2022). Skin that isn't getting enough water loses its fullness and flexibility, which makes fine lines stand out more.

For those with rosacea, a condition that causes redness and bumps, alcohol can be a real trigger. Ever get flushed after a few drinks? You might not be alone. Research suggests alcohol can widen your blood vessels, leading to facial flushing, a common rosacea symptom (Wu et al., 2015).

While alcohol doesn't directly cause acne, it can be a party pooper for those already struggling with breakouts. Alcohol can mess with your hormone balance, which can contribute to acne development. Remember how we talked about dehydration making your skin produce more oil? That extra oil creates a breeding ground for acne-causing bacteria—not exactly the kind of party favor you want!

How Cutting Back on Alcohol Can Give Your Skin a Major Glow-Up

Here's the good news: If you've been worried about how alcohol affects your skin, there's a bright light at the end of the tunnel! Cutting back on booze can lead to some serious improvements in your complexion.

First up, hydration hero status! Remember how alcohol acted like a party guest hogging all the water? Well, ditching the drinks allows your body to rehydrate properly. This translates to plumper, dewier skin with a healthy bounce—like a glowing inflatable castle ready for anything! Studies by the Australian Skin Clinics in 2020 even showed significant improvements in skin hydration for people who reduced their alcohol intake.

The next one is wrinkle reduction rhapsody! By drinking enough water, you give your skin the moisture it needs to stay flexible. This can help smooth out your skin and make fine lines and wrinkles look less noticeable, giving you a younger-looking look. Sources like the Derm Collective (Stanton, 2022) say that people who drink less, often say that their lines get better.

For those with rosacea, reducing alcohol intake can be a game-changer. Cutting back can lead to a significant improvement in your rosacea symptoms and a calmer, more even-toned complexion.

Finally, acne sufferers rejoice! Reducing alcohol consumption can be a big help. Alcohol can disrupt hormone balance and increase oil production, both of which contribute to breakouts. By limiting alcohol, you're giving your skin a fighting chance to stay clear and break out free.

Know Your Limits

Being aware of how much booze you're taking in is important, and keeping track of your drinks can help you do that. The National Institute on Alcohol Abuse and Alcoholism says that women should not drink more than one drink a day and men should not drink more than two drinks a day. On the other hand, there are many choices if you want to find alternatives to drinking or cut down a lot.

Try some tasty mocktails or cool drinks like herbal teas or sparkling water with fruit slices. And don't be afraid to talk to a doctor, therapist, or support group if you need more help. To help you on your way to living a better life, there are things you can use.

Real People, Real Results

You're not alone in this! Many people have experienced amazing skin transformations after reducing alcohol intake. Here are a couple of inspiring stories:

A Refinery29 reader shared:

"After cutting out alcohol, my skin became noticeably plumper and brighter. I also saw a reduction in redness and breakouts!" (Ollennu, 2019b).

An Allure contributor wrote:

"I quit drinking a year ago, and my skin has become clearer and smoother. I never realized how much alcohol was affecting my complexion" (Nast, 2017).

Remember, even small changes can make a big difference. By cutting back on alcohol and prioritizing hydration, you can give your skin the gift of a healthy, radiant glow!

FEELING STRESSED? IT SHOWS ON YOUR SKIN!

We all know stress can be a real drag, but did you know it can also affect your skin? It's true! Stress and skin are like frenemies—they're weirdly connected. Let's untangle this web and learn how to calm both your mind and your complexion.

The good news? Self-care is your ultimate weapon against stress (and for glowing skin!). Regularly breaking a sweat is amazing for both your mind and skin—longevity experts can swear by it. But self-care goes beyond just physical activity. It's about nurturing your emotional well-being, building strong relationships, keeping your mind sharp with activities you love, and finding ways to connect with something bigger than yourself.

Bear in mind that you don't need to do it all by yourself. If you feel like stress is winning, don't be afraid to get help from a professional. A therapist can give you the tools and advice you need to deal with stress in a healthy way, which will make you feel better and make your skin look better. In the end, a healthy mind means healthy skin.

BEAUTY SLEEP AND SKIN

Ever heard someone say, "beauty sleep" and think, "Yeah, right"? Well, guess what? You might be missing out! Beauty sleep isn't just a catchy phrase – it's a scientifically proven way to give your skin and your overall health a major boost. Let's ditch the myths and dive into the real science behind why those zzz are so important.

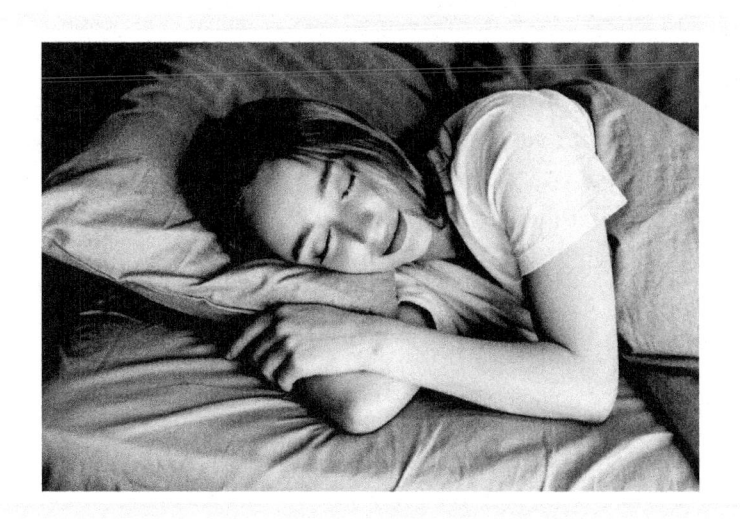

The Science Behind Beauty Sleep

While getting enough sleep might seem like a no-brainer for overall health, it's also a secret weapon for achieving radiant skin. Here's why: Science says beauty sleep isn't just a cute saying. Research from trusted sources like the Sleep Foundation, WebMD, and BBC backs this up (Suni, 2020).

Let's break it down: Sleep is a time machine for your skin! During deep sleep, your body ramps up cellular repair and regeneration. Skin cells replace themselves, fixing damage from the outside world like UV rays and pollution. This keeps your skin healthy and vibrant, with a youthful glow.

Think of sleep as a built-in, natural skincare routine. As you doze off, blood flow to your skin increases, delivering essential nutrients and oxygen. This circulation boost promotes healthy skin, leaving you with a radiant complexion that looks and feels better.

Sleep also plays a key role in keeping your skin hydrated. During sleep, your skin's natural barrier strengthens, which helps it retain moisture and avoid dehydration. This translates to supple, resilient skin with less dryness and irritation.

Finally, sleep is collagen construction time! Collagen, the protein that keeps your skin firm and elastic, gets synthesized while you snooze. This collagen production helps diminish wrinkles, fine lines, and sagging, giving you a smoother, more youthful appearance. So, the next time you hit the hay, remember you're not just resting your body, you're giving your skin a major glow-up!

Impact of Sleep Deprivation

But what happens when you skimp on sleep? Buckle up, because sleep deprivation isn't just a recipe for fatigue—it can wreak havoc on your skin too. Here's the not-so-pretty side of sleeplessness, according to sources like the Sleep Foundation and CNET.

First up, stress hormones go into overdrive. When you don't get enough sleep, your body ramps up production of stress hormones like cortisol. This can cause inflammation all over your body, which can make skin problems like acne and rashes worse. Basically, it throws your whole hormonal system out of whack, making it harder for your skin to fight off trouble.

Next, say hello to dullness and dryness. Without adequate shut-eye, your skin doesn't have enough time to repair itself from daily wear and tear. This translates to a lackluster complexion that's dry and looks, well, tired. Sleep deprivation disrupts the natural renewal process of your skin cells, leaving them weak and dull.

HOW TO CATCH THOSE BEAUTY ZZZ

Unlock the power of beauty sleep for both your skin and your overall health! Here are some super easy tips to turn your bedroom into a sleep haven and level up your shut-eye game.

First things first, ditch the salty snacks before bed. Salty foods can dehydrate you and mess with your sleep, so opt for something light and easy to digest if your tummy rumbles. Skip the heavy meals, too—you don't want to feel uncomfortable or bloated while trying to snooze.

Next, don't skip your skincare routine! Washing your face and moisturizing with gentle products before bed is a great way to signal to your body that it's time to wind down. You'll be pampering your skin while also getting ready for dreamland—win-win!

Try to get between seven and nine hours of sleep every night. Be consistent, even on weekends, with your sleep routine; this will help you immensely. Imagine it like adjusting the internal clock of your body.

Finding your perfect sleeping position is key for comfort and good sleep. Experiment with sleeping on your back, side, or stomach–whatever feels most supportive for your body and keeps your spine aligned.

Speaking of comfort, clean sheets are a game-changer! Swap them out once a week to get rid of dust, sweat, and allergens that can build up over time. Plus, there's nothing quite like climbing into fresh sheets, is there?

For dryer climates or winter months, consider a humidifier for your bedroom. It helps keep the air from getting too dry, which can irritate your skin and disrupt your sleep.

Turn off all devices at least one hour before you want to go to sleep. They make it difficult to fall asleep because the blue light they produce disrupts your body's normal circadian rhythm. Instead of reaching for your phone, try relaxing with a good book, some mild yoga, or meditation.

Make an effort to establish a relaxing nighttime pattern that your body can follow to help you wind down and get ready for sleep. If you're having trouble falling asleep, try reading a book.

Make your bedroom a haven for restful slumber! Make as little noise, light, and interruptions as possible. If you're having trouble falling or staying asleep, try using blackout curtains, earplugs, or a white noise generator to make the room more tranquil.

Last but not least, use your bedroom for sleep and intimacy only. Avoid working or watching TV in bed. This strengthens the mental connection between your bed and restfulness, making it easier to fall asleep when you crawl in.

By incorporating these tips, you can create the perfect sleep environment and unlock the power of beauty sleep for radiant skin and overall well-being. Remember, prioritizing sleep is prioritizing yourself—so sweet dreams and happy skin!

SUMMARY

This chapter has taught us that:

- You need to focus on healthy habits for glowing skin.
- Smoking accelerates wrinkles, dullness, and breakouts; quit for brighter, healthier skin.
- Alcohol dehydrates skin, worsens acne and rosacea. Cut back for brighter skin.
- Stress = skin woes. Manage stress for calmer, clearer skin.
- Beauty sleep repairs and rejuvenates skin. Prioritize sleep for a radiant look.

SEGUE

We've unlocked the power of beauty sleep, but did you know there's more to achieving a youthful glow than just catching those zzz? A consistent skincare routine, packed with the right ingredients and practices, can work wonders in slowing down the signs of aging and keeping your skin radiant for years to come.

In the next chapter, we'll delve into the world of skincare secrets for longevity. We'll explore powerful ingredients that target wrinkles, dryness, and loss of elasticity. We'll also uncover essential skincare routines tailored to different skin types. So, get ready to unlock the secrets to a timeless complexion that reflects your inner and outer beauty!

CHAPTER 4
GET TO KNOW YOUR SKIN BETTER

Have you ever glanced in the mirror and wished you'd started taking better care of your skin sooner? A recent study by Drive Research found that a whopping 67% of women over 35 harbor this very regret (Rodgers, 2023). But what if a few simple changes to your daily routine could transform that feeling into radiant confidence that lasts a lifetime?

What if you could transform that regret into a newfound confidence in your skin's health and youthful glow with a few simple changes? This chapter is your roadmap to achieving just that. We'll delve into the secrets of creating an effective skincare routine, unveil the non-negotiable role of sun protection, and explore the holistic benefits of natural and organic skincare practices. So, get ready to ditch the regrets and embrace the power of informed skincare choices!

BUILDING A PERSONALIZED SKINCARE ROUTINE

Knowing your specific skin type is the first step in developing an effective skincare routine. The same way that no two snowflakes are equal, no two people's skin is the same, and the product that moisturizes and calms your best friend's skin may actually aggravate and tighten yours. You can bring out your skin's natural glow by developing a skincare regimen that is uniquely suited to your skin type.

Here's a breakdown of the five most common skin types to help you get started:

Normal Skin

This is the holy grail—balanced, neither too oily nor too dry, with minimal visible pores. Normal skin tends to be less prone to sensitivity and blemishes, but it still needs a consistent cleansing and moisturizing routine to maintain its healthy glow.

Oily Skin

Characterized by an increased production of sebum (oil), oily skin often presents with larger, visible pores and a shiny appearance. While breakouts are a common concern, oily skin can also be quite resilient. A gentle cleansing routine with oil-free products and targeted treatments to manage shine are key.

Dry Skin

When skin is dry, it might feel tight, flaking, and itchy. Because it doesn't produce enough oil or moisture, it's more easily irritated by outside elements. For dry skin, it's important to follow a gentle washing routine and then use a rich moisturizer and moisturizing serums.

Combination Skin

This happens all the time when different parts of your face show different traits. For instance, the area around your forehead, nose, and chin may be oily, while the areas around your cheeks may be normal or dry. To achieve combination skin care, you need a mild cleanser, a moisturizer that absorbs excess oil (oil-free) for oily regions, and a heavier formula for dry parts.

Sensitive Skin

When it comes to sensitive skin, some substances or environmental factors can irritate it more than others. The skin may become red, dry, and itchy as a result. Skin that is easily irritated requires a skincare regimen that is mild, fragrance-free, and formulated with elements that relax and soothe. It is important to test new products in a limited capacity first.

As you get older, your hormones fluctuate, and even the weather can affect your skin type. Be mindful of how your skin feels and make adjustments to your routine as needed. Following this, we will get into the next section to help you develop your own routine: washing, moisturizing, and sun protection.

Take a few moments to examine your own skin before you go on to learn that. What kind of skin do you have? Is it oily? Sensitive? Perhaps a combination of two types? Make sure you know your own skin type before unlocking that skincare lottery!

IMPORTANCE OF SKINCARE ROUTINE

Did you know that taking care of your skin is more than just applying a few skincare products to your face? It's actually a self-care routine that can nourish your skin's health and even boost your mental well-being. By making skincare a priority, you're investing in your overall well-being, both physically and mentally.

You can protect your skin against the sun, acne, early aging, and other issues by sticking to a skincare routine. It has the added benefit of making your skin look healthier, brighter, and more radiant from the inside out, which is sure to lift your spirits. Taking preventative measures with your skincare routine is similar to cleaning your teeth: It will save you time and effort in the end.

And guess what? Even more so than sleeping, skincare routines are known to promote feelings of calm and contentment in the brain. Reducing stress and anxiety and increasing feelings of peace and well-being can be achieved via the practice of self-care rituals. Envision yourself washing away the stresses of the day, then delicately applying a hydrating and protecting moisturizer. Your skin will feel as good as after a little spa day!

THE ESSENTIAL STEPS OF YOUR PERSONALIZED SKINCARE ROUTINE

Now that you know what your skin type is and how important it is to stick to a schedule, we can dive into the basics of good skincare. Keep in mind that these are only the basics, and that you can tailor this plan by adding targeted remedies as required.

Cleansing

Imagine your skin is like your favorite apartment—it needs a good cleaning every now and then to truly shine! Cleansing washes away all the day's (and night's) drama—dirt, oil, makeup, and that icky pollution that loves to clog your pores and make your face look, well, less than radiant. To keep your skin glowing, think cleansing twice a day, morning and night.

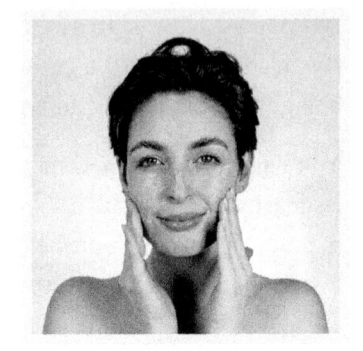

But hold on, one size doesn't fit all when it comes to cleansers. Just like you wouldn't use the same mop for hardwood floors and a plush rug, you gotta find the cleanser that works for your skin type. Got normal skin? A gentle, fragrance-free cleanser is your best friend. Bonus points if it has hyaluronic acid or glycerin for that extra hydration boost. Oily skin? To get rid of the extra oil, try using a gel or foamy cleanser. Salicylic acid can be a breakout buster, but avoid anything too harsh that dries you out.

Dry skin needs a hug in a bottle—a creamy cleanser with ceramides or colloidal oatmeal will do the trick. Combination skin? Play it safe with a gentle cleanser for your whole face, then target your oily T-zone (forehead, nose, and chin) with a separate oil-control cleanser. Super sensitive skin? Fragrance-free and hypoallergenic are your keywords. Micellar water can also be a super gentle option for those who need a little extra TLC. So, find your cleanser bestie and get ready for a brighter, happier you!

Toning

Remember that toner everyone used to rave about? It turns out, in today's skincare world, it's kind of a "maybe" step. Back in the day, toners were like the cleanup crew after washing your face, grabbing any leftover makeup or cleanser. They also aimed to balance your skin's pH level (think of it like a mood ring for your face). But guess what? Cleansers these days are pretty darn good at doing their job gently and keeping your skin's pH happy, so toners aren't a must-have for everyone.

However, if you're part of the oily-skin squad, a toner with witch hazel can be your new BFF. Witch hazel has astringent properties, which means it helps control that pesky oil and make your pores look smaller. On the other hand, if you have sensitive skin, stay clear of toners with alcohol or harsh ingredients—they'll just make your face grumpy. If you do want a little extra hydration, a toner with rosewater can be a soothing option. So, the toner debate continues, but at least you know the low-down on who might benefit from it!

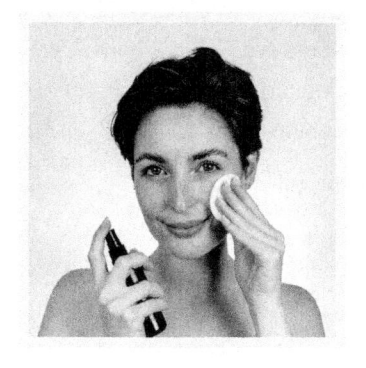

So, when you're feeling overwhelmed, your body releases special chemicals called cortisol and adrenaline. These are supposed to help you deal with danger (like running away from a hungry bear!), but they can also mess with your skin. Research shows that cortisol can lead to inflammation, which can make things like acne, eczema, or psoriasis flare up (Lankerani, 2016). Stress can also weaken your skin's natural defenses, making it easier for irritation and infection to creep in.

But wait, there's more! It's not a one-way street. Skin troubles can actually stress you out too. That's where something called psychodermatology comes in. It's a fancy way of saying that your mind and skin are super connected. Feeling stressed can show up on your skin, and vice versa.

Now, let's talk about how stress can play villain to your skin's hero story. It can trigger breakouts, worsen eczema or psoriasis, make your skin more sensitive, and even slow down wound healing. And, on top of that, chronic stress can age your skin faster by breaking down collagen and slowing down its renewal process. Not cool!

Tips to Control Acne

Feeling stressed? Don't worry, glowing skin is still within reach! Here are some super helpful tips to take control of your stress and rock radiant skin. First things first—identify your stress villains. Is it that looming work deadline, the never-ending family drama, or maybe your ever-growing to-do list that feels like it has a life of its own? Brainline.org has some fantastic resources to help you pinpoint your stress triggers.

Next, become a pro at reading your body's stress signals. Does a headache creep in, or do you feel completely wiped out? Maybe you turn into a bit of a grump, or your sleep and eating habits take a nosedive. Pay attention to these warning signs—your body is trying to tell you something!

GET TO KNOW YOUR SKIN BETTER   61

to creep in, retinol or peptides can help smooth things out.

Moisturizing

Moisture—it's kind of a skincare superhero for everyone! Whether your skin's an oil slick or a desert, keeping it hydrated is key. Think of moisturizer as a shield that traps water in your skin, making it plump, bouncy, and ready to fight off anything the environment throws at it. Plus, proper hydration keeps your skin looking younger for longer.

Here comes the exciting part: finding the best moisturizer for your specific skin type! Skin type normal? You should reach for a lightweight lotion that has SPF. Also, keep in mind that moisturizers with SPF don't really replace actual SPF. Feeling oily? Seek for a "non-comedogenic" label to identify an oil-free, lightweight moisturizer that will not clog your pores. To lock in all that moisture, dry skin longs for a heavier cream containing hyaluronic acid, ceramides, or shea butter. For combination skin apply a lighter, oil-free product to the T-zone and a thicker cream to the cheeks. Super sensitive? Find products that are hypoallergenic, fragrance-free, and formulated with soothing components such as oatmeal or aloe vera.

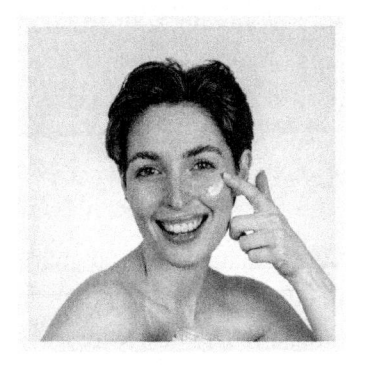

Masks

Time to put on your mask! You might think of facial masks as at-home skincare spa sessions in miniature. When applied to the skin once or twice weekly, they slather it with a potent mixture of fantastic components that address particular issues. The mask world is a veritable treasure trove of shapes, sizes, materials, and applications.

What your skin really needs will determine which mask is the best fit for it. Dealing with dry skin? Masks infused with aloe vera, honey, or hyaluronic acid will soothe parched skin. To reduce the appearance of large pores and soak up excess oil, oily skin can benefit from using a mattifying mud mask containing bentonite or kaolin clay. Also, if your skin is looking a bit lifeless, try using an exfoliating mask containing alpha hydroxy acids (AHAs) or beta hydroxy acids (BHAs) to remove dead skin cells and restore your radiance.

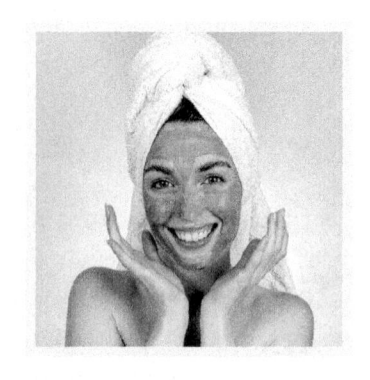

Exfoliation

To exfoliate is to give your skin a new lease on life. It removes dulling buildup of dead skin cells and oil that can cause your pores to become clogged. The best way to exfoliate varies from skin type to skin type, but exfoliating once or twice weekly will keep your skin looking healthy and radiant.

There are two main ways to exfoliate: chemical and physical. Chemical exfoliation uses products with AHAs (like glycolic or lactic acid) or BHAs (salicylic acid) to gently dissolve those dead skin cells. Physical exfoliation is more hands-on, using scrubs with sugar, oatmeal, or jojoba beads to physically scrub away the dead cells. Be gentle here—harsh scrubs can irritate your skin, so avoid them!

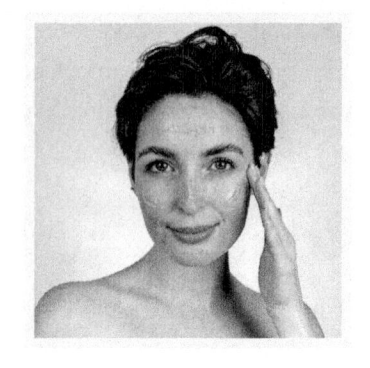

Trick: Apply a tiny amount of the product to your inner arm and wait a day or two. See if there's any redness, itching, or weirdness happening. If your inner arm gives the new product a thumbs up, then you can introduce it to your face with confidence!

MORNING AND NIGHT—YOUR PERSONALIZED SKINCARE RITUALS UNLOCKED!

Now you've got the essential skincare toolkit under your belt, let's put it all together to create your personalized morning and night routines! Here's a breakdown that keeps your skin glowing all day and night:

Morning Magic

First things first, cleanse! Wash away any leftover sleep, oil, and night cream to give your face a fresh start. Toning is optional, but if you like to use one, choose a hydrating or oil-control formula depending on your skin's needs. Just a quick spritz will do! And finally, the most important step: moisturizer with SPF! Apply a lightweight lotion with SPF 30 or higher every single morning. This is your shield that protects your skin from harmful sun damage—no excuses!

Nighttime TLC

Nighttime is your skin's chance to recharge. To remove the day's grime, oil, and makeup, start with a double cleanse. Your skin will be ready for what's to come after this. Need a more radiant complexion? Remove dull, dead skin with mild exfoliation once or twice weekly. It's also the perfect moment to use any wrinkle, acne, or concern-specific serums or treatments you may have.

Apply them after cleansing and before moisturizer. Pamper your delicate under-eye area with an optional eye cream. Finally, seal in all the goodness with a richer moisturizer than your morning lotion as you drift off to sleep. This helps your skin replenish lost moisture throughout the night. With this personalized routine, you're on your way to radiant skin, day and night!

SUN PROTECTION

While the sun might feel like a warm hug, its ultraviolet (UV) rays are a double-edged sword for our skin. Sunlight exposes us to two primary forms of ultraviolet radiation: ultraviolet A (UVA) and ultraviolet B (UVB). Skin cancer, wrinkles, and early aging are all caused by ultraviolet A (UVA) rays, which can penetrate deep into the skin's dermal layers. These rays are like sneaky villains working from the inside out. On the other hand, UVB rays are responsible for sunburns. They damage the skin's surface cells and can lead to redness, peeling, and long-term hyperpigmentation.

What does this imply for the way you normally take care of your skin? Protecting your skin from the sun is as easy as pie using sunscreen. It acts as a barrier, protecting your skin from the damaging effects of UV radiation and preserving its youthful appearance. No matter the weather, applying sunscreen first thing in the morning is an absolute must. Fine lines, wrinkles, and a lack of suppleness are all symptoms of sun damage. A healthy tan lasts longer when you use sunscreen.

The fact that clouds can't block up to 80% of UV rays shouldn't be taken for granted. Wearing sunscreen daily is a must since it provides protection even when the sky is overcast. Sunscreen is a must-have for a number of reasons, including warding off skin cancer, preventing early aging, and ensuring your skin is protected from UV radiation even on overcast days.

Sun Safety Myths Debunked!

Myth 1: Sunscreen brings on acne by blocking pores. Busted! Sunscreens nowadays won't clog pores because they aren't oil-based and don't include comedogenic ingredients. If you tend to get acne easily, it's best to stick to formulas that are classified as "non-comedogenic" for added protection.

Myth 2: Sunscreen is only for the beach. Wrong! UV rays are present even on cloudy days, so your skin needs protection year-round. Make daily sunscreen use a habit, no matter the weather.

Myth 3: A tan indicates healthy skin, right? Nope. Your skin's natural defense mechanism against UV damage is a tan. In fact, it can make you more susceptible to skin cancer and won't shield you from the sun in the future. Therefore, stop using a tanning bed and start protecting yourself from the sun.

Celebrities Get Real About Sun Protection

A lot of celebrities advocate for sun protection. It's true! These famous people rely on their flawless complexions for their careers, so they're vocal about the importance of keeping their skin safe from the sun.

Take Hugh Jackman, for example. After battling multiple basal cell carcinomas (a form of skin cancer), he's become a passionate advocate for sun safety. He urges everyone to wear sunscreen daily—and we should definitely take his advice!

Jennifer Lopez is another celebrity who swears by sunscreen. Her youthful glow is no secret, and she credits her commitment to sunscreen as a key factor. She encourages everyone to make it a daily habit, and we couldn't agree more.

And then there's Charlize Theron. This ageless beauty believes that sunscreen is the ultimate anti-aging product. She incorporates SPF into her daily routine religiously, and it definitely shows.

So, if you're looking for some inspiration to start taking sun protection seriously, look no further than these celebrity role models.

PICKING YOUR PERFECT SUNSCREEN

Protect yourself from the sun's harmful UV rays using sunscreen. However, it can be difficult to choose the correct SPF due to the wide variety of products on the market. The effectiveness of a sunscreen in blocking the sun's damaging UVB rays is indicated by its Sun Protection Factor (SPF). Therefore, more UVB protection equals a higher SPF. So, here's how it works:

- **SPF 30:** This is a great everyday option for most people. It blocks about 97% of UVB rays, which is enough for minimal sun exposure.
- **SPF 50:** Ideal for outdoor adventures or if you have fair skin. It blocks about 98% of UVB rays, offering a little more protection than SPF 30.
- **SPF 70 or higher:** The extra protection between SPF 50 and higher SPFs is pretty small. These sunscreens can also be thicker or have more ingredients, which might irritate sensitive skin.

Choosing Your Sunscreen Match

Sunscreen isn't a one-size-fits-all deal, so let's find the perfect match for your skin type!

For all you lucky ducks with normal skin, you've got options! Lotions, gels, even mineral sunscreens—the world is your oyster (or, well, your sunscreen shelf). Just pick a lightweight, oil-free formula that says "non-comedogenic" on the label. That fancy term means it won't clog your pores, keeping your skin happy and breakout-free.

Oily skin warriors, we feel you! Greasy sunscreen is the enemy. Opt for lightweight, oil-free gel sunscreens. Look for that "non-comedogenic" label again, and mineral sunscreens with zinc oxide or titanium dioxide are your best friends. They tend to be lighter and won't weigh down your skin.

Dry skin divas, hydration is key! Lotions or cream-based sunscreens are your jam. Formulas with hyaluronic acid or glycerin will give your skin an extra moisture boost, keeping it plump and healthy.

Last but not least, avoid all fragrances if your skin is sensitive. Find a mineral sunscreen that contains zinc oxide or titanium dioxide and is fragrance-free. You can safeguard your skin without worrying about irritating it thanks to these mild components.

Activity Level Also Matters

Sunscreen isn't just for beach days! Even on quick errands or commutes, SPF 30 is your daily defense against those sneaky UV rays you bump into throughout the day. But for adventures like hiking or swimming, you need a stronger shield. Grab a water-resistant SPF 50 sunscreen and reapply every 80 minutes, especially if you're sweating or swimming. Working out hard? Opt for a water-resistant AND sweat-resistant SPF 50 formula, reapplying every 40 minutes or more if you're really hitting it hard.

Bonus tip: *Lips need love too! Snag a lip balm with SPF 30 or higher to keep them protected from the sun's rays.*

NATURAL VS ORGANIC SKINCARE

Ever wonder if natural or organic skincare is the way to go? These terms get tossed around a lot, but there's a slight difference! **Natural skincare** is all about ingredients straight from nature, like calming aloe vera or luxurious shea butter. These products tend to be gentler on your skin, especially if it's sensitive, because they often skip the harsh chemicals found in some regular skincare. Think of natural ingredients as a hug for your face!

Organic skincare takes things a step further. Not only are the ingredients natural, but they're also grown without synthetic pesticides, fertilizers, or GMOs. It's a stricter standard that's better for the environment. So, why consider going natural or organic? There are some pretty cool perks:

- Natural ingredients are known to be less irritating, making them a good choice for sensitive skin.
- Many natural and organic products are eco-friendly. They might use sustainable ingredients, recyclable packaging, and have a smaller environmental footprint. It's a win-win for your skin and the planet!
- Research is showing exciting possibilities for natural ingredients in skincare. A 2023 study even suggests that certain plant extracts can help your skin stay healthy (Rodgers, 2023).

Natural doesn't always equal effective. Always choose products that work for your specific skin type. But with the abundance of natural and organic options out there, there's a good chance you can find something that nourishes your skin while being gentle and eco-friendly!

The "Natural" on Your Skincare Label

So, you're diving headfirst into natural and organic skincare—that's fantastic! But with shelves stacked high with options, how can you be sure a product is the real deal? Here are some tips to navigate those labels and unearth genuine natural or organic gems.

First, certifications like USDA Organic or COSMOS Organic are your allies. These labels guarantee the product meets specific organic standards set by independent organizations, so you know you're getting the good stuff. Next, become a label-reading pro! Look for ingredients you recognize and trust. Here are some popular natural heroes and their potential benefits:

- aloe vera, shea butter, jojoba oil (use coconut oil with caution if you're acne-prone)
- green tea extract, pomegranate extract, sunflower seed oil
- oats (perfect for sensitive skin!)
- lavender oil, licorice extract (good for redness)

Be wary of "greenwashing", though! Don't be fooled by marketing claims. If a product has a laundry list of chemicals followed by a tiny mention of "natural ingredients," it might not be as natural as it seems. Remember, even natural ingredients can be picky. Some might not be suitable for all skin types. So, before getting too excited with a new product, always do a patch test to make sure your skin agrees with it!

THREE EASY DIY RECIPES: WHIP UP YOUR OWN NATURAL SKINCARE

Ready to embrace natural skincare but want to skip the store-bought options? Look no further! Here are three simple DIY recipes using common ingredients to pamper your skin:

1. Soothing Oatmeal Face Mask

Oats are a gentle exfoliant with calming properties, perfect for sensitive skin.

Ingredients:

- 1/4 cup rolled oats, ground into a fine powder (you can use a blender or food processor)
- 2 tablespoons plain yogurt
- 1 tablespoon honey

Instructions:

1. Make a paste by mixing all the ingredients together in a bowl.
2. Once the skin is clean and dry, apply a thin coating.

3. Let it sit for 10 to 15 minutes, and then wash it off with cold water. Do a little test on your inner arm as a patch before you put it on your face. If any kind of irritation happens, stop using it.

2. Hydrating Honey Mask

Honey's natural humectant properties help draw moisture into the skin, leaving it feeling soft and supple.

Ingredients:

- 1 tablespoon raw honey
- 1 ripe avocado, mashed

Instructions:

1. Smoothly mash the avocado.
2. Add the honey and mix until smooth.
3. Use the mask on skin that is clean and dry.
4. Rinse well with lukewarm water after leaving on for 15 to 20 minutes. *Before you apply it to your face, do a patch test on a tiny section of your inner arm. Get off the product if it irritates your skin.

3. Exfoliating Sugar Scrub (for Body Only)

You will feel revitalized after using this scrub, which removes dull, dead skin cells.

Ingredients:

- 1/2 cup granulated sugar (brown sugar can be used for a gentler scrub)
- 1/4 cup coconut oil (solid, at room temperature)

- 2–3 drops of your favorite essential oil (optional—lavender or lemon are popular choices)

Instructions:

1. In a mixing bowl, mix the sugar with the coconut oil. Mix well.
2. If you are using essential oil, add it now and mix it in.
3. Scrub rough spots like elbows and knees with the scrub while you're in the shower by massaging it into wet skin in circular motions.
4. After rinsing with warm water, gently pat dry the skin.

Important Safety Reminders

- These recipes are for external use only.
- Always patch test before applying any new product to your face.
- Use fresh, high-quality ingredients.
- Store leftover homemade products in an airtight container in the refrigerator and use within a week.
- Discontinue use if you experience any irritation.

Enjoy pampering your skin with these natural DIY treats! Remember, consistency is key, so incorporate these recipes into your routine for lasting results.

SUMMARY

This chapter has taught you to

- build a personalized skincare routine based on your skin type.
- cleanse morning and night, tone (optional), and moisturize with SPF daily.

Serums

These little dropper bottles are like tiny treasure troves for your skin. Packed with concentrated ingredients like antioxidants, vitamins, and peptides, they target specific concerns like wrinkles, dark spots, or acne breakouts. Because they're so powerful, you only need a few drops after cleansing and before moisturizing.

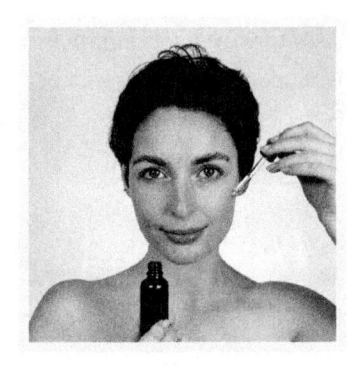

Finding the right serum is like picking out your skincare weapon of choice. For fine lines and wrinkles, serums with retinol, vitamin C, or peptides are your best bet. Battling hyperpigmentation (dark spots)? Look for serums containing vitamin C, kojic acid, or licorice root to brighten and even your skin tone. And if acne's your nemesis, serums with salicylic acid, niacinamide, or benzoyl peroxide can help clear things up.

Eye Cream

Eye spy with my little... eye cream! Your eye area has exceptionally thin skin compared to the remainder of your face, making it extremely sensitive. That's why eye creams are specially formulated to tackle concerns like dark circles, puffiness, and those pesky fine lines in this sensitive area.

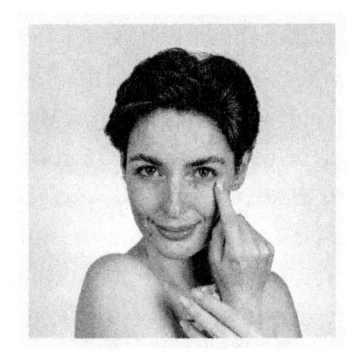

Picking the right eye cream depends on your under-eye woes. Dark circles? Look for creams with caffeine, vitamin K, or kojic acid to help brighten things up. Feeling puffy? A cooling eye cream with hyaluronic acid or cucumber extract can be your new BFF. And if fine lines are starting

- exfoliate 1-2x/week, use serums, eye cream & masks as needed.
- using sunscreen is non-negotiable! Choose SPF 30 for daily wear & SPF 50 for extended sun exposure.
- explore natural/organic options: gentle, eco-friendly, science-backed.
- look for certifications and recognize natural ingredients and their benefits.
- beware of greenwashing and patch test new products.

SEGUE

You now know that maintaining a regular skincare regimen can do wonders for your skin's condition and appearance. What if, though, you want to do more than that and fight the telltale signs of aging? We don't have to just sit back and accept the fact that we'll inevitably get fine lines, wrinkles, and a loss of suppleness as we get older. We will explore facial exercises in the upcoming chapter. So, get ready to unlock the secrets of turning back the clock (at least a little bit) on your skin!

MAKE A DIFFERENCE WITH YOUR REVIEW
UNLOCK THE POWER OF GENEROSITY

"Giving is not just about making a donation. It's about making a difference."

KATHY CALVIN

"Those who are happiest are those who do the most for others."

BOOKER T. WASHINGTON

People who give without expecting anything in return live longer, happier lives and often find success in surprising ways. So if there's a chance we can make a positive impact during our time together, let's go for it!

To make that happen, I have a question for you...

Would you help someone you've never met, even if you never got credit for it?

Who is this person, you ask? They are just like you. Or, at least, like you used to be. Someone who wants to take care of their skin, stay young, and feel great, but needs a little help to figure it all out.

Our mission is to make the secrets of skin longevity accessible to everyone. Everything we do stems from that mission. And, the only way for us to accomplish that mission is by reaching…well…everyone.

This is where you come in. Most people do, in fact, judge a book by its cover (and its reviews). So here's my ask on behalf of a struggling skincare enthusiast you've never met:

Please help that person by leaving this book a review.

Your gift costs no money and less than 60 seconds to make real, but can change a fellow reader's life forever. Your review could help...

...one more person feel confident in their skin.

...one more individual find the right skincare routine.

...one more reader discover the secret to looking youthful.

...one more person boost their self-esteem.

...one more dream come true.

To get that 'feel good' feeling and help this person for real, all you have to do is...and it takes less than 60 seconds...

leave a review.

Simply scan the QR code below to leave your review:

If you feel good about helping a faceless reader, you are my kind of person. Welcome to the club. You're one of us.

I'm that much more excited to help you achieve radiant, youthful skin faster and easier than you can possibly imagine. You'll love the tips and secrets I'm about to share in the coming chapters.

SCAN ME

Thank you from the bottom of my heart. Now, back to our regularly scheduled programming.

- Your biggest fan, Ageless Revelations

P.S. Fun fact: If you provide something of value to another person, it makes you more valuable to them. If you'd like to share the goodwill straight from another reader - and you believe this book will help them - send this book their way.

CHAPTER 5
SCULPTING BEAUTY WITH FACIAL EXERCISES

Forget six-pack abs, how about a chiseled smile? It may come as a surprise, but your face actually has muscles just like the rest of your body! The health of our faces depends on strong facial muscles, which aren't merely there for show. Having them helps us look younger, communicate our true feelings to others through laughter and smiles, and express ourselves clearly.

Picture yourself with a face that is both beautiful and expressive, which is the secret to effective face exercises! Efficiently using these muscles can enhance blood flow, strengthen muscular tone, and diminish the signs of aging. The best part? After only 20 weeks of doing face workouts every day, you can look up to three years younger, according to research from Northwestern University (Reynolds, 2018).

It may appear difficult at first to learn these exercises. Rest assured! On YouTube, you can find a great resource called FACEROBICS® that provides a number of easy routines to follow. By following their detailed instructions, you may add facial workouts to your regular regimen, which will help you look younger and more expressive than ever before.

Are you ready to stop thinking about beauty as a one-dimensional process and start utilizing your facial muscles to their full potential? This chapter will serve as a roadmap, outlining the many advantages of face workouts, presenting some basic exercises, and helping you in developing a customized program. Let's sculpt a stronger, healthier, and more expressive you, starting from the inside out!

BASICS OF FACIAL EXERCISE

Face yoga? Yep, it's a real thing! We're talking about a brighter complexion, perkier cheeks, and maybe even fewer fine lines—all without needles or fancy creams! Here's the science-y bit: Your face has a bunch of muscles (like, over 40!), and facial exercises work them out. By doing silly faces like big smiles and cheek puffs (don't worry, nobody's watching!), you boost circulation which brings fresh oxygen and nutrients to your skin. Think of it as a glow-up from the inside out.

Plus, some people say facial exercises can help your skin stay firm and bouncy by making it produce more collagen (that's the stuff that keeps your skin youthful). Over time, you might even notice fewer wrinkles and a more lifted look. Now, some folks worry about getting more wrinkles from all the exercising, but many others swear by the benefits, especially when you do it right and don't overdo it.

The best part? Face yoga is totally free and requires no equipment! Just a few minutes a day of silly moves that you can do anywhere, anytime. It might not be magic, but with a little consistency, facial exercises could be the secret weapon your skincare routine needs. So why not give your face a workout and see what happens? You might just surprise yourself!

ADVANTAGES OF FACIAL EXERCISES

Facial exercises can pump up your skin with more oxygen and nutrients, making it look plumper and glowy. Plus, they help flush out toxins and puffiness, leaving you looking fresh and de-swollen. Want sharper cheekbones and a defined jawline? Facial exercises can tone those muscles, giving you a natural contour like a superhero. And guess what? They might even help smooth out wrinkles and fine lines!

By tightening things up, those pesky lines won't be as noticeable. On top of that, facial exercises can brighten your skin by clearing out waste products, and may even help soften scars by improving blood flow. So, whether you want to say goodbye to puffiness, firm things up, or just add a little radiance, facial exercises could be the missing piece in your skincare routine. They're easy on the wallet (free!) and super simple to do, so why not give them a try and see the amazing results for yourself?

GETTING STARTED

So, are you ready to give facial exercises a go? Awesome! But before you jump in, let's make sure it becomes a habit that sticks. Here's how to kick off your facial fitness journey and get the most out of each session:

First things first: Find a chill spot where you can focus and relax. Think of it like your own personal zen zone. Wash your hands to avoid any unwanted visitors (germs) on your face, and make sure your face is clean, too. No makeup or lotion—we want your skin to move freely! Just like you wouldn't jump straight into a workout without warming up, your face needs a little prep too! Here's how to get those muscles ready to work their magic:

Give your face a relaxing spa day—at home! Use your fingertips to gently massage your forehead, temples, cheeks, and jawline in small circles. This gets the blood flowing and helps reduce puffiness, so you're ready to sculpt like a pro.

And have you ever heard of acupressure for your face? It's a thing! Gently press on some key spots like the space between your eyebrows, the middle of your cheeks, and the ends of your jaw. Hold for a few seconds each to loosen things up and get the blood pumping. Now your face is officially warmed up and ready to go.

FACIAL EXERCISES

The best part about face yoga? The moves are super easy! We're talking simple exercises that target different muscles in your face, making them stronger and bouncier. This can lead to tighter skin with fewer wrinkles—hello, youthful glow! Here are some awesome exercises recommended by face yoga experts. They each focus on specific areas, so get ready to give your whole face a workout.

The Coronation

Ready to give your whole face a lift? This exercise is a total game-changer.

1. Sit up straight and chill with your hands on your temples.
2. Now, gently push your hands up and back, like you're giving yourself a mini facelift.
3. Here comes the fun part: Open your mouth wide and stick your tongue out as far as you can, like you're trying to reach your chin.
4. Hold this silly face for five seconds, then relax. Do this five times and feel the magic happening!

The Owl

This exercise will banish those wrinkles faster than you can say "face yoga."

1. Make those finger muscles work! Create two "C" shapes with your fingers and place them gently on either side of your eyes.

2. Now comes the key part: Try to raise and lower your eyebrows while keeping your forehead completely smooth, like a total chill zone. No furrowing those brows!
3. Hold this eyebrow battle for two seconds, then relax. Repeat this awesome move six times, and watch those forehead lines fade away.

The Expressionless Face

Feeling stressed? Give your face a chill pill! This exercise is all about letting go of tension and smoothing things out.

1. Find a comfy spot and relax your whole body. Imagine you're lounging on a beach.
2. Now, try to make your face a total blank slate. No smiling, frowning, or furrowing your brows—just pure zen.
3. Hold this relaxed expression for ten seconds, then let loose. Repeat this calming move five times, and feel the stress melt away from your face!

Lick (or Kiss) the Ceiling

Targets the neck and lower face.

1. Tilt your head all the way back and look up.
2. Now, pucker your lips like you're giving the ceiling a big kiss (don't worry, it won't kiss back!). Stretch those lips out as far as you can go.
3. Hold this funny face for a few seconds, then relax. Repeat this neck and jawline toner a few times, and feel the difference.

Swan Neck

Great for toning the neck and jawline.

1. Turn your head to one side, like you're checking out what's happening over your shoulder. But don't stop there, gently tilt your head back even further, looking towards the ceiling.
2. Stretch your neck out as much as you feel comfortable, like a curious giraffe. Hold this for five seconds, then relax.
3. Repeat this neck loosener on the other side, then do three rounds on each side. You'll feel that tension melt away!

The Giraffe

This focuses on tightening the loose skin on the neck.

1. Look straight ahead and imagine your fingertips are magic wands. Place them lightly on your neck.
2. Now, slowly tilt your head back as far as feels comfortable, while gently stroking your fingertips down your neck, like you're erasing any tension.
3. Bring your head back down to your chest and repeat this soothing massage twice.

Temple Dancer Eyes

Excellent for eye muscles and reducing crow's feet.

1. Place your pointer fingers on the outer corners of your eyes, like you're gently pushing back on some sunglasses.
2. Now, open those peepers as wide as you can, like you're surprised to see your favorite celebrity. Hold this wide-eyed wonder for ten seconds.

3. Relax your eyes and repeat this awesome exercise five times. You'll be saying goodbye to tired eyes and hello to a brighter, more awake look!

The Hyoid Workout

Focuses on the lower face and chin area.

1. Open your mouth as wide as you can, like you're trying to catch a giant fly. Now, stick your tongue out as far down as you can, imagine you're trying to reach your chin with it. You might feel some tension in your throat—that's a good thing!
2. Hold this funny face for ten seconds, then relax. Repeat this triple threat move three times, and get ready to see a sharper jawline and a smoother throat!

Lion's Pose

A yoga classic that relieves tension and improves facial expression.

1. Take a big ol' sniff of air through your nose, as if you were smelling the most amazing flower ever.
2. Now, open your mouth wide, wider than you think you can, and stick your tongue out as far down as possible, like you're trying to reach your chin.
3. Here comes the fun part: Let out a mighty roar! Imagine you're a lion letting out a big yawn-roar combo. Open your eyes wide as you do this, like you're surprised by your own roar.
4. Hold this powerful pose for a few seconds, then relax your whole face. Repeat this stress-busting move twice.

The Cheekbone Lift

Helps define the cheekbones.

1. Place your fingers on top of your cheekbones, like you're giving yourself a high five.
2. Gently lift your fingers upwards, but don't let your skin move! You should feel your cheek muscles working to hold everything in place.
3. To make it even more challenging, open your mouth wide in a big "O" shape. This will really target those cheek muscles. Hold this for five seconds, feeling the burn (in a good way!).
4. Relax your face and repeat this awesome exercise ten times. Get ready to see those cheekbones getting higher and sharper with each rep!

The V

Reduces lines around the eyes and puffiness.

1. Press the tips of your middle fingers together right between your eyebrows. Now, place your pointer fingers at the outer corners of your eyes and gently press inwards.
2. Look up towards the ceiling, like you're checking out the clouds. Now comes the key part: Try to squint your eyes upwards, without furrowing your brows. Imagine you're trying to see something super tiny way up high.
3. Hold this eye-lift pose for a few seconds, then relax your face. Repeat this awesome move six times, and watch those eyelids perk up!

The Forehead Lift

Aims to reduce horizontal forehead wrinkles.

1. Place your fingers flat on your forehead, pointing towards your temples. Spread your fingers out gently, making sure they reach between your hairline and eyebrows.
2. Now, imagine you're erasing those wrinkles. Slide your fingers outwards across your forehead, applying a light but firm pressure. Think of it like smoothing out a sheet of paper.
3. Relax your face and repeat this forehead-smoothing move ten times. You'll feel the tension melt away with each swipe!

The Yummy Face Pose

Targets the muscles around the mouth and cheeks.

1. Close your lips and make the biggest, goofiest smile you can imagine. No pearly whites allowed for this one!
2. Now, puff up your cheeks like a chipmunk storing nuts for the winter. You should feel some tension in your cheeks and around your mouth.
3. Here's the tricky part: Try to smile again while holding those puffed-out cheeks. It might feel weird, but that's how you know it's working.
4. Hold this funny face for five seconds, then relax. Repeat this cheek and smile challenge five times, and get ready to see firmer cheeks and a brighter smile.

So, there you have it! These face yoga moves, recommended by all-stars like Annelise Hagen (the Yoga Face method!) and Danielle Collins, are not only super easy but can be fun too. The secret weapon to seeing results? Doing them regularly! Stick with it for a few weeks, and you might just see a glowier, tighter, and younger-looking you staring back in the mirror.

CREATING A ROUTINE

The key to rocking this face yoga thing? Doing it regularly! It's just like going to the gym—the more you show up, the better the results. But don't worry, these exercises are quick and easy, and you can totally do them while you're doing other stuff. Brushing your teeth in the morning? Perfect time for some face yoga! Watching your favorite show at night? Sneak in a few exercises during commercials. It only takes a few minutes a day, and you can multitask like a boss.

Here's a cool way to structure your face yoga week:

- **Mondays:** Start strong with exercises for your upper face, like the Forehead Lift and Temple Dancer Eyes. Bye-bye forehead lines and tired eyes, hello fresh start!
- **Tuesdays:** Time to focus on your cheeks. The Cheekbone Lift and The V will help reduce puffiness and sculpt those cheekbones.
- **Wednesdays:** Lower face workout alert! The Hyoid Workout and Lick the Ceiling will target your chin and neck, keeping things toned and tight.
- **Thursdays:** Back to the upper face. Repeat those exercises from Monday to keep those results going strong.
- **Fridays:** Full-face fiesta! Combine all the moves you learned throughout the week to maintain that overall facial awesomeness.
- **Weekends:** Relax and recharge. Skip the exercises and focus on gentle massages. This helps your face muscles recover and keeps the blood flowing.

Remember, the more you enjoy this face yoga journey, the more likely you are to stick with it. So have fun, don't stress about perfect form, and get ready to see a brighter, tighter you in the mirror!

SUMMARY

- Facial exercises, like face yoga, can tone your face and reduce wrinkles.
- Facial exercises can make you look younger.
- Facial exercises improve circulation, bringing oxygen and nutrients to your skin.
- Facial exercises can help reduce puffiness, wrinkles, and fine lines.
- Doing facial exercises just a few minutes a day is easy and can be incorporated into your daily routine.

SEGUE

Alright, you've sculpted, toned, and given your face a workout it deserves! But here's the thing—true beauty goes beyond just sculpted cheekbones and a wrinkle-free forehead. In the next chapter, we'll shift gears and explore the concept of advanced anti-aging techniques. We'll talk about laser treatments, Botox, chemical peels, their potential side effects and a lot more. So, get ready to gear up and learn the advanced tech!

CHAPTER 6
ADVANCED ANTI-AGING TECHNIQUES

Apparently, seven out of ten people are thinking about cosmetic procedures these days. Wild, right? It makes you wonder what's behind the trend. Maybe you've even considered it yourself, wondering if it's just about chasing the latest thing or if there's more to it. Well, buckle up because this chapter is all about the world of fancy skincare treatments!

We'll be diving into all the buzz-worthy stuff—laser therapy, peels, Botox, fillers—and uncovering how they're not just about erasing wrinkles, but about giving your skin a whole new lease on life. So, if you're curious about how these procedures can help you achieve a glowing, revitalized complexion, then you've come to the right place! Let's crack open these beauty secrets together and see what all the fuss is about!

LASER THERAPY

Laser therapy—sounds pretty high-tech, but it's actually simpler than it sounds and oh-so-effective for rejuvenating your skin. Imagine using light, but not just any light—the kind that's super focused and intense.

That's the core of laser therapy, which taps into the science of light to breathe new life into your skin.

Here's how it works: When the laser light is directed at your skin, it's not just shining on the surface. It's carefully calibrated to reach deeper, targeting specific issues. For example, the laser can be tuned to wavelengths that specifically interact with the pigment in brown spots or the red color in blood vessels. This precision allows the treatment to focus on just the problem areas without disturbing the surrounding skin.

This targeted approach helps stimulate your skin's natural repair processes. When the laser hits its target, it creates a controlled "injury" that, counterintuitive as it sounds, actually encourages your skin to start healing itself. Collagen formation is where the magic happens; it's the protein that gives your skin its plump, young appearance. Collagen builds up over time, making the skin smoother and firmer.

Think of it as giving your skin a gentle nudge, saying, "Hey, it's time to refresh and perk up!" It's a fascinating and effective way to get that glow back, don't you think?

Types of Lasers

Now that we've talked about how lasers rejuvenate your skin, let's dive into the different types of lasers and what each one can do for you. Trust me, there's a perfect laser out there for almost every skin concern!

First up, we have **ablative laser treatments**. These are the powerhouses of laser therapy. They work by removing the top layer of your skin, which might sound a bit scary, but it's a fantastic way to deeply resurface your skin. They're especially great for tackling deeper wrinkles, more significant sun damage, and scars. Think of them as your go-to for a major skin overhaul.

Then, there are the **non-ablative laser treatments**. These lasers are more about coaxing your skin into better shape rather than going the full demolition route. They heat up the underlying skin tissue to boost collagen production without harming the surface of your skin. These are ideal for you if you're looking for improving skin tone, texture, and fine lines, giving you that refreshed look with less downtime.

Now let's move on to something unique: **Intensive Pulsed Light (IPL)** or **Broad-Band Light (BBL)** procedures. While these do not employ actual lasers, they do use light from a spectrum that can be used to cure the skin. They work wonders for evening-out skin tone, decreasing redness, and erasing age spots. It's as if you were to impart a glow to your skin.

Finally, other forms of energy therapy such as thermal energy, radio frequency, and ultrasound must not be overlooked. Despite not being laser-based, these are frequently grouped together due to their shared characteristic of targeting the skin with energy. For a more defined and lifted appearance, they work wonders for tightening skin and reconstructing deeper tissues.

SCIENTIFIC INFORMATION HIGHLIGHTING EMERGING TRENDS AND INNOVATIONS IN LASER TREATMENTS

It's an exciting time in the world of skincare, especially when it comes to laser treatments! Advances are happening fast, offering us not only beauty solutions but also promising health benefits. Let's explore some of the cool, cutting-edge stuff that's coming our way.

First, there's some fascinating research suggesting that non-ablative fractional lasers could play a role in preventing certain types of skin cancer. Yes, you heard that right! Studies are showing that these treatments might help in reducing actinic keratosis, which are rough, scaly patches on the skin that can potentially develop into squamous cell carcinoma, a common form of skin cancer (de Vries & Prens, 2015).

It's like getting a beauty treatment that not only rejuvenates your skin but also adds an extra layer of protection against serious health issues.

And then there's acne, that age-old adversary for so many of us. New developments in laser technology are proving to be promising in the fight against those pesky breakouts. The latest trends involve using more refined laser techniques that target acne without harming the surrounding skin, reducing inflammation, and promoting faster healing. It's like giving your skin a break and letting it breathe without the constant battle with acne.

These innovations are not just about looking good—they're about genuinely promoting skin health. It's amazing to think that the same tool that helps you look your best can also protect and improve your skin's health in the long run.

TARGETED SKIN CONCERNS

Laser therapy is like a Swiss army knife for skincare—it has a tool for just about every skin concern you can think of. Let's break down some common skin issues that lasers can help address, and which types of lasers are usually called into action for each condition.

Wrinkles and Fine Lines

Ablative lasers are like a mini-bulldozer, gently smoothing away the top layer of your skin. This triggers your skin's natural healing powers, making it rebuild itself smoother and fresher. Non-ablative lasers work a bit differently. Imagine them as tiny torches that heat things up deep down. This heat tells your skin to make more collagen, which plumps things up and reduces those fine lines by making your skin more bouncy and firm—all without scraping away the surface!

Pigmentation Issues

Sunspots, age spots, uneven tone—lasers can banish them all! But the type of laser they use depends on how deep those spots go. For stubborn, deeper spots, ablative lasers are like tiny erasers, gently buffing them away. Non-ablative lasers are more like dimmers—they target the melanin (the stuff that makes those spots dark) and break it down, fading them away for a more even, brighter complexion. Either way, you'll be left with a clearer, more radiant look!

Acne and Acne Scars

Lasers can be a game-changer for acne sufferers! For those pesky breakouts, non-ablative lasers are like tiny vacuum cleaners, sucking up excess oil and zapping the bacteria that causes acne. For acne scars, ablative lasers come to the rescue. They work like mini-sculptors, gently removing the scarred tissue and encouraging your skin to grow fresh, healthy skin underneath, making those scars way less noticeable. So, smoother skin and fewer breakouts—lasers can help you achieve both!

Rosacea and Visible Blood Vessels

Rosacea and those annoying red veins? Lasers can be your new best friend! A special type called a pulsed dye laser is like a tiny sniper—it targets those blood vessels directly, shrinking them down so they're way less noticeable. This means less redness and a more even skin tone, all without harming the surrounding skin. It's a precise and effective way to get that calm, cool complexion back!

Scars and Stretch Marks

Laser therapy basically tells your skin to go into high-gear healing mode, pumping up collagen and elastin to smooth things out. Ablative lasers are like tiny sanders, buffing the surface to better blend the scar texture with your surrounding skin. Non-ablative lasers work their magic deeper down, helping your skin heal and become more elastic.

The best part? There's a laser treatment specifically designed for almost any skin concern. They're like tiny, targeted superheroes for your skin, leaving it looking and feeling healthier and more radiant!

POTENTIAL SIDE EFFECTS

While laser therapy offers some amazing benefits for rejuvenating and improving skin, like any treatment, it does come with its share of potential side effects. It's important to go into these treatments informed so you know exactly what to expect and how to take care of your skin afterward.

Redness and Swelling

After a laser session, it's common to experience some **redness and swelling**. This is your skin's natural response to the treatment, somewhat like its way of saying, "Hey, something just happened here!" This mild irritation is similar to a sunburn and usually subsides within a couple of days. During this time, keeping the skin cool and avoiding harsh skincare products can help soothe the irritation.

Skin Sensitivity to Sunlight

Post-laser treatment, your skin will be more **sensitive to sunlight**. This increased sensitivity means that stepping out without proper sun protection could lead to sunburn or further irritation. It's crucial to apply broad-spectrum sunscreen and consider wearing protective clothing, like a wide-brimmed hat, when you're outside. Think of your skin as being in a delicate state—you need to protect it like it's extra precious because, well, it is!

Peeling or Crusting

Depending on the type of laser used, especially with ablative lasers, you might notice **peeling or crusting** as the treated area heals. This isn't cause for alarm—it's just the old, treated skin making way for new skin. To manage this, keep the area moisturized and follow any specific aftercare instructions your dermatologist provides. This will help your skin heal smoothly and reduce the chance of scarring.

Pigmentation Changes

One of the more significant risks of laser therapy, particularly for those with darker skin tones, is **pigmentation changes**. This can manifest as hyperpigmentation (darker patches) or hypopigmentation (lighter patches). These effects are typically more pronounced with certain types of lasers and can be mitigated by using lasers that are appropriate for your skin type, pre-treatment skincare, and following all post-treatment care instructions carefully.

BEFORE AND AFTER THE PROCEDURE

Getting ready for a laser treatment isn't just about marking your calendar for the big day. There's a bit you'll need to do beforehand to make sure your skin is prepped and ready to receive all the benefits laser has to offer. And of course, taking care of your skin after the procedure is just as crucial to ensure you get those fabulous results. Let's break it down:

Before the Procedure

Put on as much sun protection as you can find. This is something you must do whether or not you are undergoing laser therapy, but it is absolutely necessary if you are. Use a high-SPF sunscreen and stay out of the sun for a few weeks leading up to your treatment if you can. This lessens the likelihood of pigmentation problems after treatment.

Next, put a pause on certain skincare products that might irritate the skin. Products containing retinol, glycolic acid, or benzoyl peroxide should be avoided for a week or two before your session. Your skin should be in its most calm, natural state to handle the laser effectively.

It's also a good idea to stay hydrated and maintain a healthy diet leading up to the procedure. Hydrated skin responds better to laser treatment, healing faster and more effectively.

After the Procedure

Post-treatment care is all about soothing and protecting. Keep the treated area clean and moisturized with gentle products recommended by your dermatologist. Continue to avoid direct sunlight and use a broad-spectrum sunscreen to protect your new skin.

Avoid picking at any peeling or flaking skin—let it come off naturally. This is part of the healing process, and keeping your hands off will prevent scarring.

AFTERCARE FOR OPTIMIZED RESULTS

After your laser treatment, taking care of your skin is super important to get the best results and that post-laser glow. Here's how to be a champion at aftercare:

Your skin might feel a bit like it got a sunburn—totally normal and usually only lasts a few hours. To soothe things down and reduce any redness or puffiness, grab a cool compress and gently pat your skin.

For the first day or two, ditch your usual skincare routine and keep things simple. Use gentle, fragrance-free cleansers and moisturizers. Your doc might even recommend special aftercare products to help your skin heal even faster. Avoid anything harsh or scrubby—your skin needs a vacation from those for a while!

Moisturizer is your new BFF! Dry skin is itchy and uncomfortable, and it can slow down healing. Slather on a rich, fragrance-free moisturizer to keep your skin soft and happy. Drinking plenty of water is also a win-win. It hydrates your skin from the inside out, which helps it heal faster and keeps you glowing all over. Sun protection is a must after laser treatment! Think SPF 30 sunscreen, reapplied every two hours when you're outside. Sun exposure can darken those treated areas, so suit up and protect that precious new skin!

Also, give yourself a break from heavy workouts for the first few days. Sweating can irritate your skin, and pools or saunas are breeding grounds for bacteria, which you definitely don't want after a laser. Relax, recover, and hit the gym when your skin's feeling good as new. Don't skip your follow-up appointments with your dermatologist! These check-ups are important to make sure your skin is healing beautifully, and you're getting the results you wanted.

SHARON'S STORY

Sharon's journey with laser therapy encapsulates perfectly the transformative power of this treatment. Just before her wedding, an event where everyone wants to look their absolute best, Sharon decided to go for an ultra-fractional laser treatment. She was aiming to tackle some stubborn skin issues that had bothered her for years, and wanted to glow on her big day.

Sharon had some sun damage, uneven skin tone, and noticeable indications of aging before she started the treatment. These are common concerns that many of us share, making her story so relatable. The decision wasn't made lightly, as the timing was crucial—she needed to be fully healed and looking her best in time for her wedding.

After her treatment, the results were nothing short of spectacular. Sharon noticed significant improvements in the texture and tone of her skin. The treatment effectively diminished fine lines and lightened age spots, giving her a refreshed and rejuvenated appearance. Her skin not only looked smoother but also felt firmer.

On her wedding day, Sharon looked radiant. The confidence she felt from her improved appearance was evident in her smile and the sparkle in her eyes. This before-and-after scenario really highlights how impactful, well-timed, and expertly executed laser treatments can be. It's not just about the aesthetic enhancement—it's about how these changes make you feel. Knowing that you are perfect just the way you are on your most important day can make all the difference, as Sharon's story shows.

CHEMICAL PEELS

Want to give your skin a fresh start? Look no further than chemical peels! Think of it as a restart button for your face, buffing away the old, tired layers to reveal the glowy, youthful skin hiding underneath.

Here's how it works: A special chemical solution is applied to your skin, and it gets to work by gently dissolving the top layers. Don't worry, it's a controlled process! This exfoliation encourages your skin to grow a brand new, healthier layer. The result? Smoother, clearer skin with fewer wrinkles and an even tone—basically, a total radiance upgrade!

Chemical peels can seriously tackle a variety of concerns. They can soften fine lines and wrinkles, fight acne breakouts, fade dark spots, and even minimize scars. Plus, they're a great option for anyone who wants a brighter, more youthful appearance without going under the knife. Chemical peels also give your collagen production a boost, which is like adding natural plumpers to your skin.

Therefore, a chemical peel could be the answer to your prayers if you're seeking a way to restore the skin's natural radiance. And the good news is, these treatments are constantly getting better. Recent studies show that chemical peels are more effective and comfortable than ever before (Khunger & Chanana, 2022).

For example, a study published on found that new peels are designed to be gentle and cause minimal downtime, while still delivering amazing results for all kinds of skin types and concerns (Șoimița Emiliana Măgerușan et al., 2023). Whether you're battling acne, uneven skin tone, or fine lines, there's likely a peel out there that can help!

Another study dermatology looked at glycolic acid peels specifically for treating melasma (stubborn brown patches on the face) (Sharad, 2013). The results were fantastic—people's skin tone and texture improved significantly. Plus, this study showed that glycolic acid peels are well-tolerated, making them a great option for long-term skincare routines.

These studies show that chemical peels are a powerful tool in a dermatologist's toolbox. They can be customized to address various skin concerns, and they keep getting better and better. Chemical peels are a great option to consider if you want to revitalize your skin and get a healthy shine!

Types of Chemical Peel

Chemical peels come in all strengths, from gentle refreshers to deep-down rejuvenators. Think of them like choosing the right cleaning tool for your home—you wouldn't use a power washer for dusting the shelves! Here's a quick guide to the three main types of peels to help you find your perfect match:

Light Chemical Peels

These peels are like a super gentle buffing session. They use mild acids to whisk away only the top layer of your skin. This is a great option for concerns like fine lines, acne scars, uneven tone, or just some general dryness. The best part? Minimal discomfort and barely any downtime—you can practically bounce right back to your day! The results might be subtle at first, but with a few treatments, your skin will be noticeably fresher and brighter.

Medium Chemical Peels

Going a bit deeper, medium peels target both the top and middle layers of your skin. They use slightly stronger acids to tackle concerns like sunspots, wrinkles, freckles, and uneven pigmentation. They can also smooth out rough texture. Expect some tingling or stinging with this peel, and the recovery takes a few days. Your skin might turn red and swell a bit, and then form crusts that flake off over a week or so.

Deep Chemical Peels

Deep peels are the heavy-duty option. They use powerful ingredients to reach the deepest layers of your skin. These are great for addressing deep wrinkles, sun damage, scars, and even precancerous growths. Because they're so intense, they require anesthesia and a longer recovery time—think two weeks for healing, with some redness lingering for a few months. However, the results are dramatic and long-lasting—you might only need one treatment for a serious skin transformation!

Potential Risks and Side Effects

Chemical peels, while awesome, can have some side effects, especially if not done by a pro. During recovery, it's common to experience some redness, dryness, or a bit of stinging or burning. Sensitive skin might get a little puffy or extra red too.

There are also some rarer, but more serious risks, like scarring, infections, or changes in your skin color—this is especially true for deeper peels. People with darker skin tones also have a higher chance of getting dark spots after the peel.

To avoid these not-so-desirable effects, here's the key: Follow all the instructions your doctor gives you before and after the peel, and make sure you choose a qualified professional to do the treatment.

What to Expect

Chemical peels are like hitting the rewind button on your skin—hello, fresh start! During the treatment, you might feel a little tingle as the peel works its wonders. Afterwards, your skin might be a bit red and start to peel—that's just the old layers saying goodbye!

To keep that post-peel glow going strong, here's the secret: Baby your skin! Use a gentle cleanser, pile on the moisturizer (seriously, hydration is key!), and avoid the sun like it's yesterday's news. Think of the sun as your skin's worst enemy right now. By following these steps, your skin will stay smooth, clear, and radiant for a long time after the peel. So, you can ditch the dullness and embrace a brighter, younger-looking you!

BOTOX FOR WRINKLE REDUCTION

Botox—it's everywhere in the beauty world, a brand that everyone must have heard of once in their life. But what exactly does it do? Botox, short for botulinum toxin (say that ten times fast!), is like a tiny messenger blocker for your muscles. When injected in specific areas, it stops the nerves from telling those muscles to flex. This makes the muscles relax and soften, which smooths out wrinkles caused by all that squinting and frowning—think forehead lines, crow's feet, and those deep lines between your brows.

But that's not all Botox is for! Also, it is a miracle cure for several health issues. For people with chronic migraines, excessive sweating, or muscle issues like neck spasms, Botox can be a game-changer. It can even help with crossed eyes or uncontrollable blinking. Whether you're aiming for a smoother look or managing a medical condition, Botox is a minimally invasive option that works for 3–6 months. That versatility is why so many people love it—it keeps you looking and feeling your best!

Case Studies

Science is catching up with what many people already know—Botox is pretty amazing! Recent studies are confirming how effective it can be for both beauty and medical concerns. One study by the National Institutes of Health looked at Botox for chronic migraines. Guess what? People who got regular Botox injections had way fewer headaches (Shaterian et al., 2022)! This is exciting news for migraine sufferers, as it could be a long-term solution to those awful head throbs.

Another study focused on Botox's wrinkle-reducing superpowers. The results? Botox definitely smooths out those lines and wrinkles, and most people who got it were much happier with their appearance (Satriyasa, 2019). So, whether you're looking for a younger-looking you or relief from migraines, Botox seems to be a double win!

Potential Risks and Considerations

Botox is pretty awesome, but like anything else, it can come with some minor bumps in the road. For example, you might get a little bruise or feel some discomfort at the injection site—nothing major, but worth mentioning. There's also a chance of headaches or, in rare cases, the treated area might droop a bit, especially if you don't go to a pro. These side effects are usually temporary, but they definitely emphasize why choosing a qualified and experienced doctor is key.

Here's the thing: Botox results can vary, especially when it comes to cosmetic treatments. That's why a personalized plan is super important. Make sure you find a reputable provider who will listen to your goals and create a treatment plan that's just right for you. By prioritizing safety and going to a pro, you can minimize risks and maximize those Botox benefits—win-win!

What to Expect

Botox treatments are pretty quick and easy—usually just a few minutes in and out! No need for anesthesia, so you can get your zap and get on with your day. To minimize bruising, skip the alcohol and anti-inflammatory meds for a few days beforehand.

After your injections, stay upright for a few hours and avoid rubbing the treated areas—you don't want the Botox playing peek-a-boo in unintended places! You'll start to see the results in a few days, and they can last for months. Regular touch-ups can keep your smooth, refreshed look going strong. Most importantly, follow your doctor's aftercare instructions to the T. This will ensure the best results and minimize any chance of bumps in the road. Easy as that!

DERMAL FILLERS FOR VOLUME RESTORATION

Say goodbye to wrinkles and hello to a younger-looking you! Dermal fillers are a popular choice for people who want to fight the signs of aging without going under the knife. Dermal fillers are like tiny plumpers that fill in those wrinkles and add volume back to your face. This plumps things up and gives you a smoother, more youthful appearance. Think of it as putting bounce back into your skin!

Types of Dermal Fillers

There are several types of dermal fillers, each suited to different needs and areas of the face. Understanding the differences between them can help determine which is the best option for specific concerns:

Hyaluronic Acid (HA)

Hyaluronic acid (HA) is a superstar among fillers because it's already naturally found in your skin. This means it's super safe and effective for filling in wrinkles and plumping up those areas that have lost volume. HA fillers can tackle concerns like scars, wrinkles, and lines by smoothing things out and adding volume. They're popular for plumping lips, adding fullness to cheeks, and even filling in hollows under the eyes. The best part? The results are temporary, lasting anywhere from 6 to 12 months. This is because your body naturally absorbs the HA over time. So, it's like a mini-makeover with built-in expiration date—no commitment required!

Calcium Hydroxylapatite (CaHA)

Need a more heavy-duty filler for those deeper wrinkles? CaHA (say that one five times fast!) is your friend. This type of filler is a bit thicker than HA and is naturally found in your bones. It acts like a double threat—filling in those deep lines and wrinkles, and also telling your skin to produce more of its own natural plumping collagen. This makes CaHA fillers a great choice for adding volume to your cheeks and sculpting your facial contours. The best part? They can last up to 18 months, so you can enjoy that youthful look for a longer stretch!

Polymethyl Methacrylate (PMMA)

PMMA is a long-lasting filler option for those deeper wrinkles and folds. Think of it as a semi-permanent solution for those stubborn lines you just can't seem to banish. Made with a special collagen gel and tiny spheres, PMMA fillers provide immediate support and scaffolding for your own natural collagen production. Over time, your skin starts pumping out more collagen to fill things in even more. This makes

PMMA fillers a great choice for tackling nasolabial folds (those lines that run from your nose to your mouth) and other deep wrinkles. Keep in mind that PMMA is on the longer-lasting side—results can stick around for up to five years!

Poly-L-lactic Acid

PLLA is another filler superstar, and it's all about stimulating your own natural collagen production. This means it doesn't just fill in wrinkles, it tells your skin to get busy making its own plumpers over time! PLLA is a popular choice for tackling deeper wrinkles and folds, and the results can last for a whopping two years or more. Think of it as a long-lasting investment in your youthful look—like a wrinkle-fighting superhero! An added bonus? PLLA is biodegradable, so it eventually gets broken down by your body.

Human Fat

Fat grafting is like borrowing from your own body for a natural-looking makeover! Doctors take fat cells from another area, like your tummy or thighs, purify them, and then inject them into wrinkles or areas that need more volume, like your cheeks. It's more involved than other fillers, but the results can be amazing and long-lasting—sometimes even permanent!

Potential Risks and Considerations

Dermal fillers can do wonders for your youthful look, but like anything else, there can be some minor bumps in the road. It's common to experience some redness, swelling, or bruising at the injection site—nothing major, but worth mentioning. These usually disappear within a few days.

There are also some rarer, but more serious risks, like allergic reactions, infections, or uneven results. In very rare cases, something called vascular occlusion can happen, where the filler accidentally blocks a blood vessel. This can be serious, so it's important to choose a qualified professional who knows how to minimize these risks.

Here's the key: Always go to a certified and experienced doctor who is knowledgeable about the specific fillers and techniques they're using. A good provider will answer all your questions and make sure you're a good candidate for fillers in the first place.

What to Expect

Dermal fillers are a pretty quick and easy way to refresh your look. In and out in about 30 minutes, depending on what areas you're targeting. You might feel a pinch during the injection, but they often use numbing cream to minimize discomfort. After the treatment, it's normal to see some swelling or bruising, but don't worry, that usually fades within a few days.

Here's what you can do to help your face heal: Take it easy on the exercise for a day, and avoid super hot or cold temperatures. The best part? You'll see results practically right away, and they can last for months or even years, depending on the type of filler used.

SUMMARY

This chapter has taught you to:

- Ditch wrinkles! Lasers zap away fine lines and age spots, leaving you glowing.
- Buff and brighten! Chemical peels remove dull layers for smoother, younger-looking skin.
- Relax and rejuvenate! Botox smooths wrinkles caused by frowning and even helps with migraines.
- Plump it up! Dermal fillers add volume to wrinkles and restore a youthful appearance.
- Consult a pro! Safe and effective cosmetic procedures require a qualified professional for best results.

SEGUE

Injected your way to a smoother, younger you? Now let's talk about keeping it that way—naturally! While lasers, peels, and fillers work wonders, self acceptance can be a powerful tool to sculpt your true beauty, delaying the signs of aging and complementing your newfound glow. Flip the page and discover how a little makeup tips can go a long way in keeping your youthful look in tip-top shape!

CHAPTER 7
EMBRACING NATURAL BEAUTY

"I can't think of any better representation of beauty than someone who is unafraid to be herself."

EMMA STONE

Accepting and celebrating your individuality—flaws and all—is the key to genuine beauty. That feeling of confidence that comes from being happy with who you are. How often have you felt an irresistible pull toward someone whose contagious laugh or quirky sense of humor made the room feel more lively? Or maybe someone who fights for their values, no matter how unpopular they may be? Being authentic is like a magnet, it draws in and inspires. That's the magic we're going to tap into in this chapter!

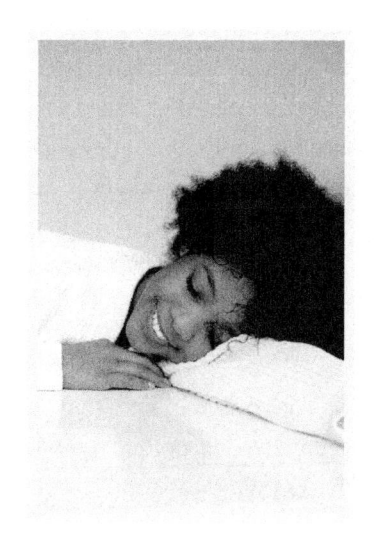

We'll explore ways to boost your self-love, learn some simple tricks to highlight your natural features, and even pick up makeup tips that enhance your true self, not hide it. Basically, this chapter is your cheerleader guide to unleashing your inner and outer sparkle every single day. Here's to being you, beautifully and unapologetically!

WHO ARE YOU?

Have you ever stopped to think about how you see yourself? Imagine yourself standing in front of a mirror, but instead of focusing on your physical reflection, look deeper. What are your strengths? What are your quirks? Do you smile at the person looking back, or do you flinch at perceived flaws?

This internal reflection, this perception of who you are, is your self-image. It shapes how you navigate the world, how you interact with others, and ultimately, how happy you feel. But sometimes, that self-image can be distorted, filled with harsh judgments and unrealistic expectations. This is where self-acceptance and self-love come in.

Self-acceptance is one of those journeys that looks different for everyone, yet it's foundational to genuine happiness and a robust sense of self-esteem. It's about recognizing your worth, embracing your entirety, both strengths and flaws, and giving yourself a little grace. It means seeing yourself as deserving of happiness and respect, no matter your mistakes, achievements, or what you see in the mirror. Think of Michelle Obama, a powerful woman who wasn't afraid to embrace her natural curls, defying conventional beauty standards and inspiring countless others to do the same.

Self-love is the next step. It's about cherishing who you are and celebrating your unique qualities. Take Viola Davis, an award-winning actress who once spoke about overcoming self-doubt to find her voice. Her journey of self-love empowered her to achieve incredible success.

Learning to accept and love yourself isn't always easy. It takes time, effort, and maybe even a few stumbles along the way. But the rewards are immeasurable. By embracing yourself, you unlock a sense of confidence and inner peace that allows you to shine brightly.

Still, it's not always easy to embrace ourselves completely. The constant barrage of ideal and successful people in our media might distort our perception of ourselves by drawing attention to our weaknesses rather than our strengths. When we're always comparing ourselves to others, it can be hard to accept ourselves.

Why is it so tough? Maybe it's because it makes us feel exposed to admit our true selves, flaws and all. Sometimes, we have to face painful facts, like mistakes we've made in the past or parts of our looks we've been taught are "less desirable." The exciting part, though, is that wonderful things begin to happen as soon as we begin to lower these walls, as soon as we begin to treat ourselves with the same love and kindness that we would show to a close friend. The way we feel about ourselves changes.

A kind, honest space inside ourselves is what self-acceptance is all about, not being rude or having an ego. It means telling yourself, "Hey, I'm doing my best, and that's enough." It helps you feel better about yourself and boosts your confidence. So, how about we start that journey today? But first, let's take a look at some studies.

THE SCIENCE BEHIND SELF-ACCEPTANCE

Turns out, liking yourself is a total game changer. Research shows that accepting yourself and feeling good about who you are is like magic shields protecting your mental health (Godwin, 2022). Well, studies also say self-acceptance helps you bounce back easier (Kashdan, 2021). Another study found that people with higher self-esteem tend to be happier and deal with setbacks like a champ (Baumeister et al., 2003). They don't let rejections get them down for long and come back stronger.

The coolest part? Some research suggests that simply accepting yourself might be even more important than feeling super awesome about yourself all the time (K, 2023). It means being okay with your flaws (we all have them), and that can lead to way fewer mental health struggles in the long run.

Basically, these studies are like a big high five, saying *"Hey, you! Be kind to yourself, and you'll be happier and healthier for it!"* So, let's all work on accepting ourselves exactly as we are. It's the first step to feeling fantastic!

CULTIVATING SELF-ACCEPTANCE

Building yourself up is like building a fort—it takes some time and effort, but the end result is pretty awesome! Accepting yourself, totally and completely, isn't something that happens overnight. It's a long haul, and like any adventure, it requires a few tools and tricks.

First up: forgiveness. We all mess up sometimes, but holding onto those mistakes is like carrying a heavy backpack—it weighs you down. Acknowledge what happened, understand it doesn't define you, and then let it go! Think of it like letting go of a deflated balloon—it just floats away. Be kind to yourself, just like you would be to a friend who made a mistake.

Treat yourself with kindness, not criticism! That nagging voice in your head that loves to point out your flaws? Time to mute it! When things get tough, or you notice something you're not crazy about, instead of beating yourself up, offer yourself some compassion. Talk to yourself like you would your best friend—with understanding and encouragement.

Sometimes our brains like to play mean tricks on us. We get stuck focusing on the negative, dwelling on past "failures" or things we wish we did differently. Instead, try to see those experiences as stepping stones, lessons that helped you grow. It's all about flipping the script!

You are amazing, and don't forget it! Take some time to celebrate your wins, big and small. Aced that presentation? Totally rocked that new outfit? Give yourself a mental high five! Reminding yourself of your strengths and accomplishments is a surefire way to boost your confidence.

Surround yourself with people who make you feel good! Having a positive support system is like having a cheering squad in your corner. These are the people who lift you up, believe in you, and remind you of how awesome you are, especially when you're feeling down.

Last but not least, gratitude! Take a moment each day to appreciate the good stuff in your life, big or small. Maybe it's your comfy PJs, that delicious cup of coffee, or a good laugh with a friend. Keeping a gratitude journal is a great way to train your brain to focus on the positive. There will be ups and downs, but by following these tips and being kind to yourself, you'll be well on your way to building a strong and positive self-image. You've got this!

BUILDING SELF-CONFIDENCE

Confidence isn't just a feeling, it's like a winner cape you wear all the time! It's knowing you've got what it takes, no matter what. Here are some ways to build that inner confidence and keep it strong:

- Stop the comparison trap first. Social media can make it seem like everyone else has their life perfectly together, but trust me, that's not always the real story. The only person you should compare yourself to is... yourself yesterday. Focus on how far you've come and celebrate your own unique journey.
- Take care of yourself, mind and body! Treat yourself like the awesome person you are. Getting enough sleep, eating healthy, and doing things you enjoy all add up to feeling good about yourself.

- Do stuff you rock at! When you're doing things you're good at, it's like a built-in confidence booster. It reminds you of your skills and what you're capable of achieving.
- Challenge yourself to grow. Stepping outside your comfort zone might sound scary, but it's a great way to discover hidden talents and surprise yourself with what you can do. Every challenge you overcome is a confidence building block!
- Be your own cheerleader. The way you talk to yourself matters. Instead of negative self-talk, swap it out for positive pep talks. The more you tell yourself you can do it, the more you'll believe it!
- Affirmations roll. These are short, positive statements that remind you of your strengths. Repeating them to yourself can help drown out those self-doubts and build up your confidence muscles.
- It's okay to say no. Setting boundaries is a sign of strength, not weakness. Knowing when to say no protects your time and energy, which helps you feel more empowered and confident.
- Set goals you can crush! Don't set yourself up for failure with impossible goals. Set small, achievable goals that you can celebrate along the way. Each accomplishment, big or small, is a win for your confidence piggy bank!

ENHANCING NATURAL FEATURES WITH MAKEUP

For ages, makeup has been a way for people to play up their natural beauty and show off their unique style. Ever feel like your eyes could be a little more "pop"? A touch of mascara can do wonders. Maybe you want a flawless base for your selfies? Foundation can help you achieve that airbrushed look. The point is, makeup is there to boost your confidence and let you put your best face forward, however you define "best."

Makeup isn't about hiding who you are—it's the other side of the coin, freedom of expression. It's a box of artistic tools for your face, letting you create any look you can imagine. Feeling bold and dramatic? Go for a smoky eye and a bold lip. Want something softer and whimsical? Play with pastel colors and glittery accents. There are no rules, just endless possibilities to express yourself and create a look that reflects your unique personality.

And guess what? Tons of people use makeup! Studies show that the average woman uses a bunch of beauty products every day, and a whole lot of them feel more confident when they're wearing makeup, especially with eye products like mascara (Mafra et al., 2022). That confidence can spill over into everything you do, from rocking a presentation at work to slaying your next social gathering.

Here's the coolest part, makeup isn't about completely changing your face. It's more about highlighting your natural features, the stuff that makes you, unique. Whether you go for a subtle look or a full-on glam beat, it's all about expressing yourself and having fun. So, whether you want a little extra oomph for your self-esteem, want to polish your look for work, or just want to experiment and get creative, makeup is a powerful tool to add to your beauty bag!

CONTOURING TECHNIQUES

Contouring is a transformative makeup technique that can enhance your natural features, sculpt your face, and highlight your best assets according to your unique face shape. Whether you're aiming to slim, shorten, lengthen, or balance your features, understanding how to contour specifically for your face shape can make a significant difference. Here's a simple guide to get you started:

Contouring for Different Face Shapes

Round Face

For those with round faces, the goal is to create definition and elongate the face. Apply a contour shade around the edges of your face, starting from the temples and curving down to just below the cheekbones and along the jawline. This creates shadows that visually sculpt the face, making it appear more angular and oval.

Square Face

If you have a square face, contouring can help soften the angular edges to enhance your natural features. Apply contour on the sides of your forehead and below your cheekbones, starting from your ears and ending in the middle of your cheeks. This technique helps narrow the appearance of the forehead and jaw, giving a more rounded look to the face.

Oval Face

Oval faces have a natural balance, so the contouring goal here is to maintain proportion. Apply a subtle shadow under your cheekbones and along the hairline to refine the natural contours of your face.

Heart Face

For heart-shaped faces, apply contour under your cheekbones, starting from your ears and tapering to the ends of your lips. Add a little contour to the forehead along your hairline to balance the narrower chin.

Eye Makeup for Different Eye Shapes

Contouring doesn't stop at your cheeks; your eyes can also be enhanced through specific techniques tailored to their shape:

Almond Eyes

Enhance almond eyes by using eyeshadow to create a subtle gradient from the lash line, blending outwards. Darker shades at the outer corners will emphasize the natural upsweep.

Round Eyes

To elongate round eyes, focus dark shadows on the outer corner and extend slightly beyond the edge of the eye. This creates a more cat-like shape, giving the illusion of wider, more dramatic eyes.

Hooded Eyes

Apply darker shades in the crease to add depth. Light shimmery shades on the brow bone can also help lift the eye area, countering the droopiness that hooded lids might give.

Monolid Eyes

Use gradient shading by applying darker colors close to the lash line and blending lighter shades upwards toward the eyebrow, creating dimension and depth.

Makeup Techniques for Different Lip Shapes

Lips are a central feature of expression, and enhancing them can change the character of your face:

Thin Lips

For thinner lips, overline your natural lip line slightly with a lip liner close to your natural color and fill in with a light, creamy lipstick to add fullness.

Full Lips

Celebrate full lips by using bold colors. You can apply a bit of gloss in the center of the lower lip to enhance their volume even more.

Uneven Lips

If your lips are uneven, use a lip liner to correct and balance their shape before applying lipstick. Choose matte shades to minimize attention to any asymmetry.

Blush Application for Different Face Shapes

Blush can also be used strategically to enhance your face shape:

Round Faces

Apply blush slightly to the side of the center of your cheeks and sweep it towards the ears. This helps create a more defined face shape.

Square Faces

Softly apply blush on the cheekbones, blending towards the temples to soften the angles of your face.

Oval Faces

For oval faces, apply blush directly on the cheekbones and blend outwards to enhance the natural contours.

Heart Faces

Apply blush on the bottom of your cheeks and sweep upward toward the ear lobe. This technique helps balance the width of your forehead with your narrower chin.

Understanding these techniques and using them in a way that works for you will help your makeup look its best and bring out your natural beauty in the best way possible. Remember that blending is the key to perfect contouring. Make sure there are no harsh lines and that the change from one shade to another is smooth.

NATURAL MAKEUP LOOK

Achieving a natural makeup look is all about letting your real beauty shine through without too much fuss. Choosing the right products is key to this effortless, "barely there" appearance, and it starts with finding shades and formulas that complement your natural skin tone beautifully.

Foundation

Opt for a lightweight foundation or a tinted moisturizer that matches your skin tone perfectly. This will help even out your complexion without masking it. The goal is to look like you're not wearing any foundation at all. If you have good skin, you might even skip foundation entirely or just use a bit of concealer where needed.

Blush and Bronzer

For blush, go for a color that mimics your natural flush. Peachy or light pink shades tend to look soft and subtle, enhancing your complexion in a sun-kissed, natural way. A touch of bronzer applied lightly under the cheekbones, along the temples, and under the jawline can add warmth and a hint of contour without looking too dramatic.

Eyes and Lips

When it comes to your eyes, a swipe of brown or taupe eyeshadow and a coat of clear or brown mascara can lift your lashes while keeping things minimal. For lips, a tinted balm or a lipstick in a nude or pink shade close to your natural lip color will add just the right touch of polish.

SIMPLE EVERYDAY MAKEUP ROUTINE

Creating a simple, everyday makeup routine that enhances your natural beauty without feeling overdone is all about using the right products and techniques. Here's a step-by-step guide to achieving a fresh, minimal makeup look perfect for daily wear:

1. Prime for Your Skin Type

Start with a primer that suits your skin type. If you have dry skin, look for a hydrating primer; for oily skin, a mattifying primer works best. Primer helps create a smooth base and ensures your makeup lasts longer throughout the day.

2. Reach for a Light-Coverage Base

Apply a light-coverage foundation, BB cream, or tinted moisturizer that complements your skin tone. Starting in the middle of your face and working your way outward, apply it using your fingers, a beauty sponge, or a brush. The idea is to make your skin tone look more uniform while yet achieving a sheer, undetectable layer of coverage.

3. Conceal in the Areas That Need More Coverage

If you have any blemishes or dark circles, apply a lightweight concealer in a shade that closely matches your skin. Use a small brush or your fingertip to blend the concealer gently where needed.

4. Swipe on Some Bronzer

To bring warmth to your face, lightly dust bronzer along your hairline, under your cheekbones, and along your jawline. Use a fluffy brush for a natural, sun-kissed effect.

5. Add Cream Blush and Highlighter

To apply cream blush, pick one that looks like your natural flush, and then use your fingers to dab it over your cheekbones and mix it up toward your temples. Use a cream highlighter on your cheeks, brow bones, and down the bridge of your nose to give your face a soft glow.

6. Apply Mascara and Neutral Eye Makeup

For the eyes, keep it simple: A swipe of neutral eyeshadow on the lids can define your eyes subtly. Finish with a coat of black or brown mascara to open up your eyes and make your lashes look naturally fuller.

7. Fill in Your Brows

Your eyes will be framed and emphasized by neatly trimmed eyebrows. To fill in sparse areas, follow your brow's natural shape with a brow pencil or gel. Use a little touch because the look is meant to be natural.

8. Add a Hydrating Lippie

Complete your look with a swipe of hydrating lip balm or a tinted lip balm for a hint of color. This adds a fresh, polished touch to your natural makeup look without feeling heavy.

This routine is all about enhancing your features subtly and effectively, giving you a polished look that's perfect for everyday activities. Remember, the key to a natural makeup look is to use products sparingly and blend well. This way, you achieve a beautiful look that feels as good as it looks!

SUMMARY

- Shine bright, be you. Confidence starts with self-acceptance.
- Ditch the masks, embrace your flaws. True beauty is all you.
- Makeup? A tool to enhance, not hide.
- Contour your face, conquer your day.
- Natural beauty, effortless glow! Your everyday makeup routine.

SEGUE

We've unlocked the secrets to unleashing your inner and outer radiance, but true beauty starts with a healthy foundation—literally! In the next chapter, we'll dive into essential skincare routines to keep your skin glowing for years to come. Get ready to learn how to protect your skin for the long haul!

CHAPTER 8
PROTECTING YOUR SKIN FOR THE LONG HAUL

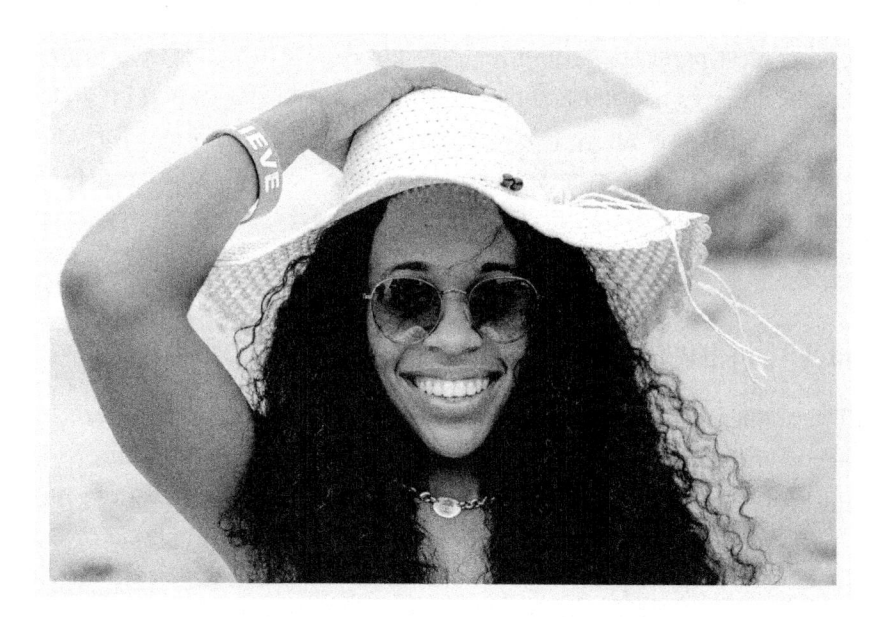

How often do you think about the influence that your sun protection routines have? Do you prioritize frequent skin checks for your health? This chapter is devoted to helping you understand why it's important to check your skin often, how to avoid skin cancer, and what you can do to protect yourself from environmental hazards. Our mission is to provide you with the tools you need to take charge of your skin's health in the modern world by teaching you how to prevent damage and keep it healthy.

ROUTINE SKIN CHECK-UPS

Skin check-ups are like getting your car serviced every year—a routine pitstop to ensure everything's running smoothly and catch any potential problems before they become major headaches.

These check-ups aren't just about skin cancer, though that is a big one! Dermatologists can also spot signs of other skin woes, like eczema or funky acne breakouts, and nip them in the bud before they get out of hand. Early detection is key, especially with skin cancer, where catching it early makes treatment way more successful.

The coolest part? By getting regular skin exams, whether by a pro or by checking yourself at home, you become a total skin expert on yourself. You'll know all your moles, marks, and what's normal for your skin, making it super easy to spot anything new or different. These check-ups could literally be lifesavers, and even if not, they'll keep your skin happy and healthy.

HOW TO PERFORM A SELF-EXAMINATION

The sooner you catch something, the easier it is to zap it away! To become a skin sleuth, grab a full-length mirror and a handy mirror for those tricky spots. Find a bright room (think sunshine streaming in) and get comfy. Start by checking your face, nose, lips, and ears. Use that hand mirror to peek at your scalp (part your hair with a comb for a good look) and then move on down to your arms, hands, chest, back (bend over for this one!), legs, and even your nether regions (don't worry, everyone does it!). Stand on your tiptoes to see the sides of your shoulders, and sit down to check your legs thoroughly.

Moreover, take pictures of your skin so you can compare them later. The more you know about your moles, marks, and freckle constellations, the easier it is to spot any new visitors. If you see something new, a mole that's changed, or a weird patch of skin that just won't heal, hightail it to a dermatologist. They're the skin experts. Regular self-exams paired with check-ups from the pros are your ultimate defense for keeping your skin happy and healthy. So, grab your mirrors, channel your inner detective, and give your skin some TLC!

WHEN TO SEEK PROFESSIONAL HELP

While self-exams are a great way to stay informed, there are times when a dermatologist's expertise is crucial. Here's when to consider scheduling an appointment:

Firstly, any changes in your moles warrant a visit. This includes shifts in size, shape, color, or border. New moles or any that appear different from the others are also cause for concern. Remember the "ugly duckling" rule—if a mole sticks out from the crowd, it's best to get it checked. Additionally, persistent skin issues like redness, dry patches, or wounds that just won't heal could signal conditions like psoriasis or eczema. Unexplained itchiness or pain shouldn't be ignored, either. A dermatologist can investigate the cause and recommend the appropriate treatment.

Early detection is key when it comes to skin health. If you notice any new lesions or changes in existing ones, particularly if they bleed, ooze, or crust over, schedule a visit with a dermatologist. These can sometimes be indicators of skin cancer. Do not hesitate to consult a dermatologist; they will be able to alleviate your concerns, identify the root of the problem, and design a unique treatment plan just for you. After all, your skin is your largest organ, and it deserves the best care possible!

SKIN CANCER PREVENTION

Sun safety might not be the first thing on your mind, but hear me out! Skin cancer is actually super common, and even though it's often preventable, a lot of us are missing key info on how to stay safe in the sun. Whether you're a total beach bum or just catching rays on your daily commute, understanding skin cancer is a big deal for your health.

Here's the lowdown, skin cancer happens when stuff called UV rays (from the sun or tanning beds) mess with your skin cells' DNA. This mix-up makes the cells grow out of control, forming a bunch of abnormal cells, aka skin cancer. Melanoma, the most dangerous kind, is one of several varieties of cancer; the others include basal cell carcinoma and squamous cell carcinoma.

Common Risk Factors

Sun exposure is the main culprit behind skin cancer, especially for those who spend a lot of time soaking up the rays or have a history of bad sunburns, particularly when they were younger. But there are other things that can up your risk too:

- People with fair skin, light hair, and light eyes naturally have less melanin, which is like sunscreen made by your body. So, they tend to burn easier and need extra sun protection.
- If skin cancer runs in your family, you might be more prone to it due to your genes.
- Ever hit up the tanning salon? Those UV rays aren't any friendlier to your skin than the sun's.
- Living in a place with intense sunshine or high altitude means stronger UV rays, so be extra cautious.
- Having a ton of moles or freckles, or skin that burns or freckles instead of tanning, can also be risk factors.

Skin Cancer Statistics

Skin cancer is definitely something to keep an eye on. The American Academy of Dermatology says nearly 20 people in the US die from melanoma every single day, which is pretty scary (American Academy of Dermatology Association, 2022). Also, sunburn lovers beware! Studies show getting burned just five times can double your risk of melanoma (MoleMap Team, 2021). But the good news? If you catch it early, the survival rate for melanoma jumps to a whopping 99% (Cleveland Clinic, 2021)! So, basically, prevention and catching it early are your best bets to keep your skin healthy.

Signs and Symptoms of Skin Cancer

Skin cancer is no joke, but knowing the signs can make a big difference. Here's what to keep an eye out for:

- If a new mole pops up or a sore just won't heal after a few weeks, get it checked by a doc.
- Existing moles are your friends, but if they start changing their shape, size, or color, that's a sign to get them looked at. Remember the ABCDE rule: Asymmetry (wonky shape), Border irregularity (ragged edges), Color that's not uniform (like a patchy mess), Diameter bigger than 6mm (about the size of a pencil eraser), and Evolving size, shape, or color (growing or changing like a chameleon).
- Any strange changes to your skin, like scaly patches, weird itching, or new growths you weren't expecting, deserve a visit to the doc to be safe.

Preventative Measures

Spotlighting skin cancer might sound scary, but it isn't really. It's mostly preventable with a few tweaks to your daily routine.

Apply sunscreen first. Always, even on overcast days, apply a broad-spectrum sunscreen with an SPF of 30 or greater. Always reapply after sweating or water play, and at least every two hours. Arm yourself with sun protection gear, including long-sleeved shirts, slacks, hats with wide brims, and sunglasses. You should seek out shade as much as possible between 10 a.m. and 4 p.m., when the sun's rays are at their fiercest. Sleep it off—tanning beds are a skin cancer magnet! Your skin tone is lovely the way it is, so don't try to change it.

On top of sun protection, there are other cool things you can do for your skin that are pretty easy to squeeze into your day. Eating a balanced diet with lots of antioxidants is like giving your skin a built-in shield against the sun's rays. Think fruits and veggies high in vitamin C and E—those are your best bets. Staying hydrated is another superstar for your skin. When you're well-watered, your skin stays plump and resilient, ready to face whatever the environment throws at it, sun or not. So basically, by doing these simple things every day, you're not just protecting your skin, you're giving your whole body a major high five!

Remember, these small changes can make a big difference. By taking steps now to lower your exposure to UV rays, you're investing in your long-term health. Win-win!

ENVIRONMENTAL PROTECTION

Our skin is kind of like a special suit, protecting us from the outside world. But just like any suit, it can get worn down over time. Here's how some sneaky environmental villains that can damage your skin and how to fight back!

Gross Germs

Public places are crawling with icky germs, and touching your face after grabbing a subway pole can lead to irritation and breakouts. Washing your hands often and keeping your fingers off your face are your best weapons here.

Air That Steals Moisture

Dry climates and cranked-up heaters can suck the moisture right out of your skin, leaving it feeling parched. Fight back with a humidifier—it'll add moisture to the air, keeping your skin plump and happy.

Pollution Problems

City air is full of pollutants that can damage your skin. Antioxidants in skincare products can act like a shield, while washing your face at night removes those yucky particles that settle on your skin during the day.

Weather Woes

Both super hot and super cold weather can mess with your skin. Cold air can make it dry and cracked, while hot weather can lead to breakouts. Dressing for the weather and adjusting your skincare routine with the seasons is key.

To keep your skin looking and feeling its best, consider using sunscreen (always!), products with antioxidants, and moisturizers. Drinking plenty of water also helps your skin stay strong against environmental attacks. Little things like using a humidifier, washing your face regularly, and using the right moisturizer can make a big difference!

SUMMARY

This chapter has taught you:

- Sunshine? Yes. Skin damage? No. Unveiling sun protection strategies.
- Skincare goes beyond SPF. Protect your skin from daily environmental aggressors.
- Pollution, dryness, extreme weather—fight back for healthy, resilient skin.
- Your skin's best defense is a multipronged approach. Keep exploring!
- From sun to smog, we've got your skin covered. Learn how to shield it all!

SEGUE

We've established the importance of protecting your skin's physical health, but true beauty goes deeper. The next chapter explores the powerful connection between mental well-being and a radiant inner glow. In Mental Well-Being and Timeless Beauty, we'll discover how self-care, mindfulness, and a positive outlook can enhance your natural beauty and leave you feeling confident from the inside out.

CHAPTER 9
MENTAL WELL-BEING AND TIMELESS BEAUTY

Pause and think about everything you've been through. When you're under pressure, how does your skin typically respond? Does your skin's condition seem to be affected by your emotions? Have you seen any patterns? This chapter will go into more detail on the critical relationship between your skin and your mind, how taking care of one can benefit the other, and why your skin can benefit greatly from a holistic approach to health.

THE CONNECTION BETWEEN MIND AND SKIN

Ever notice your skin acting up when you're stressed? It turns out there's a real connection between your mind and your skin! A study showed there are a few ways stress and skin can play off each other (Koo & Lebwohl, 2001). Following is a breakdown of this study:

First, there are conditions like eczema or psoriasis that might not be caused by stress but can definitely get worse when you're feeling overwhelmed. It's like stress throws gasoline on those skin issues. On the flip side, there are mental health conditions where people might actually hurt their own skin. Think hair pulling or picking at their skin—

these can be signs of something deeper going on mentally (Koo & Lebwohl, 2001).

And lastly, the study talks about how bad skin problems can sometimes lead to feeling down or anxious. For example, someone with severe acne might feel self-conscious and withdraw from social stuff, which can affect their mental health. So, basically, it's a two-way street: Stress can mess with your skin, and skin problems can mess with your mind (Koo & Lebwohl, 2001). That's why taking care of both your mental and physical health is super important. By keeping your stress levels in check and taking care of your skin, you're giving your whole well-being a big boost!

MANAGING STRESS FOR HEALTHIER SKIN

Managing stress is not just good for your mental health—it's essential for keeping your skin glowing and healthy too. Here are some practical ways you can reduce stress and, in turn, help your skin look its best.

Mindfulness and Meditation

These are powerful tools for calming the mind and reducing stress. Spending even just a few minutes each day in meditation can help lower cortisol levels and reduce the overall stress load on your body.

Try guided meditations or mindfulness apps to get started; they provide simple, step-by-step instructions that make it easy to incorporate meditation into your daily routine.

Yoga

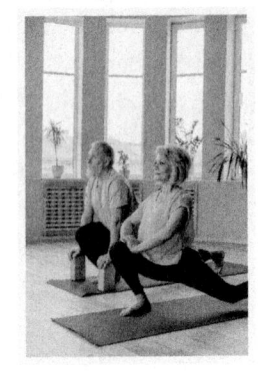

Combining physical movement with breath control and meditation, yoga is a comprehensive practice that can significantly reduce stress. Whether it's a gentle Hatha session or a more vigorous Vinyasa flow, yoga helps release tension stored in the body and soothes the mind.

Regular Exercise

Physical activity releases endorphins, natural mood lifters, which can help alleviate stress. Activities like walking, cycling, or swimming are not only great for your health but also give you a break from the daily grind.

Establish a Routine

A regular routine can significantly reduce stress by removing uncertainty about what you need to do and when. Include skin-nourishing practices in your routine, such as applying a moisturizer daily and ensuring you get enough sleep each night.

Connect With Nature

Spending time in green spaces can lower stress levels and improve your mood. Even a short walk in a park can help clear your mind and refresh your skin.

Adding these habits to your routine will not only help you deal with stress, but they will also help your skin from the inside out. Remember that your skin usually feels better when you feel good in your mind.

EMOTIONAL RESILIENCE AND BEAUTY

Emotional resilience plays a pivotal role in maintaining not just our inner health, but also our outer beauty. It's the armor that helps us manage life's ups and downs without letting them leave a mark on our appearance. When we're emotionally resilient, we're better equipped to handle stress and anxiety, which are often directly reflected in the health of our skin.

Take the story of Jenna, for instance. After years of battling severe acne, which flared up during stressful periods, Jenna began incorporating mindfulness and yoga into her daily routine. As she developed greater emotional resilience, her flare-ups became less frequent and her skin started to clear. This transformation wasn't just skin deep; Jenna felt more vibrant and confident, which radiated from her as visibly as her smoother skin.

Then there's Mark, who suffered from eczema that was exacerbated by his high-stress job. His skin condition improved significantly when he adopted stress management techniques and pursued a more balanced lifestyle. Mark's journey to better skin was a testament to how managing emotional health can lead to tangible changes in one's physical appearance.

These stories highlight a profound truth: Cultivating emotional resilience can lead to a healthier and more attractive appearance. Practices like regular exercise, sufficient sleep, and maintaining social connections don't just build our mental and emotional health; they help us look our best. By fostering emotional resilience, we empower ourselves to face life's challenges with a steady mind and a glowing complexion.

INTEGRATING MENTAL WELLNESS INTO SKINCARE ROUTINES

Integrating mental wellness into your skincare routine can transform what might feel like a mundane daily task into a rejuvenating self-care ritual. Here's how you can blend these practices to not only care for your skin but also soothe your mind:

Meditative Breathing

As you begin your skincare routine, take a moment to practice deep, meditative breathing. With each application of cleanser, moisturizer, or serum, take slow, deep breaths. Inhale the calming scents of your products and use the rhythmic movements of applying creams or serums as a focus point for your breath. This practice can help center your thoughts and reduce stress, making your skincare routine a grounding experience.

Gratitude Practice

Turn your skincare routine into a moment of gratitude. As you look at yourself in the mirror, think of three things you are grateful for about your body or your day. This positive reflection can boost your mood and self-esteem, contributing to a healthier mental state.

Mindful Observation

Pay close attention to the texture of your skin and the feel of each product you apply. Notice the sensations as you massage your skin—how each stroke feels, the coolness of a cream, or the softness of a foam. This mindfulness can help you connect with the present moment and leave you feeling refreshed and relaxed.

SUMMARY

- Stress can lead to breakouts, dullness. Learn how your mind impacts your skin.
- Chill vibes, glowing skin! Manage stress with meditation, yoga, and nature walks.
- Inner strength, outer beauty. Emotional resilience keeps your skin healthy and radiant.
- Transform your routine with mindful breathing and gratitude.
- Mind-skin connection—nurture your well-being for a healthy, confident you.

KEEPING THE GAME ALIVE

Now you have everything you need to unlock the secrets of skin longevity, it's time to pass on your newfound knowledge and show other readers where they can find the same help.

Simply by leaving your honest opinion of this book on Amazon, you'll show other skincare enthusiasts where they can find the information they're looking for, and pass their passion for skincare forward.

Thank you for your help.

The quest for ageless beauty is kept alive when we pass on our knowledge – and you're helping us to do just that.

Scan here to leave your review on Amazon:

CONCLUSION

We've flipped the final page, but the story of your radiant skin is just beginning! This book wasn't just a science lesson (although, that antioxidant stuff was pretty cool, right?). It was your personal guide to unlocking the secrets of lifelong skin health.

We discussed the magic of a holistic approach—how good food, mindful routines, and a healthy lifestyle become your skin's ultimate dream team. You learned about the power of antioxidants, crafted a personalized routine, and gained the knowledge to make informed choices about your skin's care.

But this isn't a one-time read. This book is your trusted companion, ready to guide you as your skin's needs evolve throughout life. Remember, your skin is as unique as your fingerprint, a living canvas that tells your story. It deserves a personalized approach that grows and changes with you.

So, it's time to grab your highlighter and rewrite the ending! Don't be afraid to experiment with the tips and tricks we explored. Whip up a DIY face mask, discover the magic of facial massage, or delve deeper into the world of natural ingredients. Remember, the most important ingredient is your curiosity and a playful spirit!

The real secret to timeless beauty? Self-love. Forget chasing fleeting ideals of youth. It's about embracing the skin you have, every laugh line, every sun-kissed memory etched onto your beautiful canvas. It's about appreciating the resilience of your skin, its ability to heal and transform.

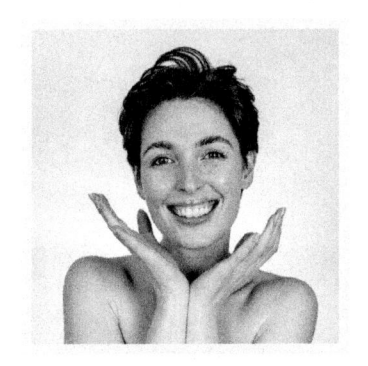

Skincare with self-love transforms your routine from a chore to a daily ritual of appreciation. As you cleanse, tone, and moisturize, take a moment to acknowledge the incredible organ you're nurturing. Your skin is your largest and most dynamic protector, a bridge between you and the world. Show it some love!

Because when you feel good in your own skin, it shows. Confidence radiates from within, adding a natural glow that no product can replicate. So, prioritize your mental and emotional well-being, too. Get enough sleep, chase joy, surround yourself with positive people. Let your inner light shine through!

Remember, this skin health journey is a conversation, not a monologue. Share your discoveries with others! Maybe you found a hidden gem of a natural product or mastered the at-home facial. Sharing your knowledge empowers others and fosters a community of glowing skin warriors!

And in that case, we're thrilled to invite you to join the exclusive **Ageless Revelations Community** on Facebook! In this group of like-minded folks, you can

- access exclusive resources, checklists, and tools to support your journey.
- share experiences and insights with fellow skincare enthusiasts.

- find motivation and support from others on the same path.
- connect with a community that celebrates healthy skin and a positive outlook on life.

Join the **Ageless Revelations Community** today and let's keep the conversation glowing! Thank you for joining me on this adventure! It's been an honor to be your guide through the science and art of nurturing your natural beauty. May your skin forever reflect the care, knowledge, and love you invest in it, today and always.

Now, go forth and conquer your skincare goals! You've got this, glow getter!

GLOSSARY

Antioxidants: Molecules that neutralize harmful free radicals, which can damage skin cells and contribute to wrinkles and other signs of aging.

Ceramides: Fatty molecules that help maintain the skin's barrier function, keeping it hydrated and protected from environmental damage.

Collagen: A protein that provides structure and support to the skin, giving it a plump and youthful appearance. Collagen production naturally declines with age.

Elastin: Another protein that gives skin its elasticity and allows it to snap back after stretching. Like collagen, elastin production decreases with age.

Epidermis: The outermost layer of the skin, responsible for providing a barrier against the environment.

Exfoliation: The process of removing dead skin cells from the surface of the skin, promoting cell turnover and a brighter, smoother complexion.

Hyaluronic Acid: A naturally occurring substance in the skin that helps it retain moisture, keeping it plump and hydrated.

Inflammation: The body's natural response to injury or infection. Chronic low-grade inflammation can contribute to skin aging.

Oxidation: A chemical reaction involving free radicals that can damage skin cells.

Photoaging: The premature aging of the skin caused by exposure to ultraviolet (UV) radiation from the sun.

Retinol: A form of vitamin A that promotes cell turnover and collagen production, helping to reduce wrinkles and improve skin texture.

SPF (Sun Protection Factor): A measure of a sunscreen's ability to protect against UVB rays, which are the primary cause of sunburn and contribute to skin cancer.

UVA Rays: A type of ultraviolet radiation that penetrates deeper into the skin than UVB rays. UVA rays contribute to wrinkles, loss of skin elasticity, and hyperpigmentation.

UVB Rays: A type of ultraviolet radiation that damages the outer layers of the skin, causing sunburn and increasing the risk of skin cancer.

Wrinkles: Lines and folds in the skin caused by a breakdown of collagen and elastin, sun damage, and other factors.

REFERENCES

American Academy of Dermatology Association. (2022, April 22). *Skin Cancer.* Aad.org; American Academy of Dermatology Association. https://www.aad.org/media/stats-skin-cancer

antigoneelectra. (2021, January 14). *When I was smoking m....* Reddit. https://www.reddit.com/r/scacjdiscussion/comments/kx34fx/comment/gj8h94b/?utm_source=share&utm_medium=web2x&context=3

Australian Skin Clinics. (2020, December 20). *What alcohol is doing to skin.* Australian Skin Clinics. https://australianskinclinics.com.au/blog/what-alcohol-is-doing-to-your-skin/

Baumeister, R. F., Campbell, J. D., Krueger, J. I., & Vohs, K. D. (2003). Does High Self-Esteem Cause Better Performance, Interpersonal Success, Happiness, or Healthier Lifestyles? *Psychological Science in the Public Interest, 4*(1), 1–44.

Bowe, W. P., & Pugliese, S. (2014). Cosmetic benefits of natural ingredients. *Journal of Drugs in Dermatology: JDD, 13*(9), 1021–1025; quiz 26-27. https://pubmed.ncbi.nlm.nih.gov/25226001/

Canadian Lung Association. (2016). *There are 4000 chemicals in every cigarette | the lung association.* Lung.ca. https://www.lung.ca/lung-health/smoking-and-tobacco/whats-cigarettes/there-are-4000-chemicals-every-cigarette

Cherney, K. (2018, March 7). *Zinc for acne: cystic, scars, OTC products, and more.* Healthline. https://www.healthline.com/health/beauty-skin-care/zinc-for-acne#oral-or-topical-zinc

Cleveland Clinic. (2021, June 21). *Melanoma: Symptoms, stages, diagnosis, treatment & prevention.* Cleveland Clinic. https://my.clevelandclinic.org/health/diseases/14391-melanoma#:

Culliney, K. (2023, February 22). *Wrinkles, fine lines and eye bags top global skin concerns in 2022.* Cosmeticsdesign-Europe.com. https://www.cosmeticsdesign-europe.com/Article/2023/02/22/Revieve-report-shows-wrinkles-fine-lines-and-eye-bags-biggest-skin-care-concerns-in-2022-globally

de Vries, K., & Prens, E. P. (2015). Laser treatment and its implications for photodamaged skin and actinic keratosis. *Current Problems in Dermatology, 46,* 129–135. https://doi.org/10.1159/000367958

Godwin, J. (2022, November 6). *Let's talk about... self acceptance.* Let's Talk about Mental Health. https://letstalkaboutmentalhealth.com.au/2022/11/06/self-acceptance/

Jennings, S. (n.d.). *Sharon's Story: I got ultra fractional laser right before my wedding.* Mybeautybunny.com. Retrieved May 23, 2024, from https://mybeautybunny.com/sharons-story-i-got-ultra-fractional-laser-right-before-my-wedding/

K, Ó. (2023, February 6). *Self-Acceptance: The road to a happier life.* Medium. https://orlakenny.medium.com/self-acceptance-the-road-to-a-happier-life-e4f2b4bce6ad

REFERENCES

Kashdan, T. (2021, October 20). *What helps us bounce back from adversity – Confidence? Grit? Self-Compassion? Hope?* Todd Kashdan. https://toddkashdan.com/what-helps-us-bounce-back-from-adversity-confidence-grit-self-compassion-hope/

Khunger, N., & Chanana, C. (2022). A perspective on what's new in chemical peels. *Cosmoderma, 2*, 14. https://doi.org/10.25259/csdm_5_2022

Koo, J., & Lebwohl, A. (2001). Psycho dermatology: the mind and skin connection. *American Family Physician, 64*(11), 1873–1878. https://pubmed.ncbi.nlm.nih.gov/11764865/

Lankerani, L. (2016, April 22). *How the stress hormone cortisol is damaging your skin*. Westlake Dermatology®. https://www.westlakedermatology.com/blog/how-stress-is-damaging-your-skin/#:

Li, S., Cho, E., Drucker, A. M., Qureshi, A. A., & Li, W.-Q. (2017). Alcohol intake and risk of rosacea in US women. *Journal of the American Academy of Dermatology, 76*(6), 1061-1067.e2. https://doi.org/10.1016/j.jaad.2017.02.040

Mafra, A. L., Silva, C. S. A., Varella, M. A. C., & Valentova, J. V. (2022). The Contrasting Effects of Body Image and self-esteem in the Makeup Usage. *PLOS ONE, 17*(3). https://doi.org/10.1371/journal.pone.0265197

Manalo, D. (n.d.). *7 ways drinking water helps improve skin: Pure luxe medical: Medical Spa*. Www.pureluxemedical.com. https://www.pureluxemedical.com/blog/7-ways-drinking-water-helps-improve-skin#:

Mary. (2023, March 17). *What happened to my body ater I quit smoking*. Patient's Lounge. https://patientslounge.com/mental-health/What-Happens-to-your-Body-when-you-Quit-Smoking

Michalak, M., Pierzak, M., Kręcisz, B., & Suliga, E. (2021). Bioactive compounds for skin health: A review. *Nutrients, 13*(1), 203. https://doi.org/10.3390/nu13010203

MoleMap Team. (2021, April 27). *How many sunburns does it take to get skin cancer? | MoleMap Australia*. Www.molemap.net.au. https://www.molemap.net.au/skin-cancer/sunburn#:

Nast, C. (2017, November 24). *I quit drinking for a month and it totally transformed my skin*. Allure. https://www.allure.com/story/i-quit-drinking-alcohol-and-my-skin-cleared-up

National Institute on Alcohol Abuse and Alcoholism. (2023). *Drinking levels defined*. Nih.gov. https://www.niaaa.nih.gov/alcohol-health/overview-alcohol-consumption/moderate-binge-drinking

News in Health. (2017, September 8). *Sun and skin*. NIH News in Health. https://newsinhealth.nih.gov/2014/07/sun-skin

Ogawa, Dr. R. (n.d.). *International Journal of Molecular Sciences*. Www.mdpi.com. Retrieved April 29, 2024, from https://www.mdpi.com/journal/ijms/special_issues/scar_biology

Ollennu, A. (2019a, February 9). *I stopped drinking for 30 days — & my skin got so much better*. Www.refinery29.com. https://www.refinery29.com/en-us/cutting-out-alcohol-skin-benefits

Ollennu, A. (2019b, February 9). *I stopped drinking for 30 days — & my skin got so much better*. Www.refinery29.com. https://www.refinery29.com/en-us/cutting-out-alcohol-skin-benefits

Reynolds, G. (2018, January 10). Facial exercises may make you look 3 years younger. *The New York Times*. https://www.nytimes.com/2018/01/10/well/move/facial-exercises-may-make-you-look-3-years-younger.html#:

Rodgers, E. (2023, August 24). *Skincare statistics and trends in 2023*. Www.driveresearch.com. https://www.driveresearch.com/market-research-company-blog/skincare-statistics-and-trends/

Satriyasa, B. (2019). Botulinum toxin (Botox) A for reducing the appearance of facial wrinkles: a literature review of clinical use and pharmacological aspect. *Clinical, Cosmetic and Investigational Dermatology, Volume 12*(12), 223–228. https://doi.org/10.2147/ccid.s202919

Sharad, J. (2013). Glycolic acid peel therapy – a current review. *Clinical, Cosmetic and Investigational Dermatology*, 6, 281. https://doi.org/10.2147/ccid.s34029

Sharma, N., Chaudhary, S. M., Khungar, N., Aulakh, S. K., Idris, H., Singh, A., & Sharma, K. (2024). Dietary Influences on Skin Health in Common Dermatological Disorders. *Cureus*. https://doi.org/10.7759/cureus.55282

Shaterian, N., Shaterian, N., Ghanaatpisheh, A., Abbasi, F., Daniali, S., Jahromi, M. J., Sanie, M. S., & Abdoli, A. (2022). Botox (OnabotulinumtoxinA) for Treatment of Migraine Symptoms: A Systematic Review. *Pain Research and Management, 2022*, e3284446. https://doi.org/10.1155/2022/3284446

Șoimița Emiliana Măgerușan, Hancu, G., & Rusu, A. (2023). A Comprehensive Bibliographic Review Concerning the Efficacy of Organic Acids for Chemical Peels Treating Acne Vulgaris. *Molecules, 28*(20), 7219–7219. https://doi.org/10.3390/molecules28207219

Stanton, C. (2022, May 16). *Your skin health before and after quitting alcohol*. Derm Collective. https://dermcollective.com/skin-health-before-and-after-quitting-alcohol/

Story, E. N., Kopec, R. E., Schwartz, S. J., & Harris, G. K. (2010). An Update on the Health Effects of Tomato Lycopene. *Annual Review of Food Science and Technology, 1*(1), 189–210. https://doi.org/10.1146/annurev.food.102308.124120

Suni, E. (2020, October 23). *How sleep works: Understanding the science of sleep*. Sleep Foundation. https://www.sleepfoundation.org/how-sleep-works

Sutaria, A. H., & Schlessinger, J. (2019, October 25). *Acne Vulgaris*. National Library of Medicine; StatPearls Publishing. https://www.ncbi.nlm.nih.gov/books/NBK459173/

Vaillancourt, K., Ben Lagha, A., & Grenier, D. (2021). A green tea extract and epigallocatechin-3-gallate attenuate the deleterious effects of irinotecan in an oral epithelial cell model. *Archives of Oral Biology, 126*, 105135. https://doi.org/10.1016/j.archoralbio.2021.105135

Wu, S., Li, W.-Q., Qureshi, A. A., & Cho, E. (2015). Alcohol consumption and risk of cutaneous basal cell carcinoma in women and men: 3 prospective cohort studies. *The American Journal of Clinical Nutrition, 102*(5), 1158–1166. https://doi.org/10.3945/ajcn.115.115196

Yahya Mahamat-Saleh, Al-Rahmoun, M., Gianluca Severi G, Reza Ghiasvand, Veierod, M. B., Saverio Caini, Palli, D., Edoardo Botteri, Sacerdote, C., Fulvio Ricceri, Lukic,

M., Sánchez, M. J., Pala, V., Tumino, R., Chiodini, P., Amiano, P., Colorado-Yohar, S., María-Dolores Chirlaque, Ardanaz, E., & Bonet, C. (2022). Baseline and lifetime alcohol consumption and risk of skin cancer in the European Prospective Investigation into Cancer and Nutrition cohort (EPIC). *International Journal of Cancer*, *152*(3), 348–362. https://doi.org/10.1002/ijc.34253

Printed in Great Britain
by Amazon